New frontiers in cancer therapy

Non-myeloablative stem cell transplantation (NST)

Published by Darwin Scientific Publishing Ltd

New frontiers in cancer therapy

Non-myeloablative stem cell transplantation (NST)

Edited by

Sergio Giralt
Bone Marrow Transplant Unit, University of Texas M. D. Anderson Cancer Center, Houston, TX, USA

and

Shimon Slavin
Department of Bone Marrow Transplantation and Cancer Immunotherapy, Hadassah University Hospital, Jerusalem, Israel

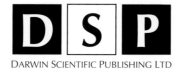
DARWIN SCIENTIFIC PUBLISHING LTD

Published by **Darwin Scientific Publishing Limited**
Abingdon, Oxfordshire, United Kingdom

© Darwin Scientific Publishing Ltd 2000

First Published 2000

ISBN 1-903557-00-3

British Library Cataloguing-in-Publication Data

A catalogue record for this book is available from the British Library.

Printed in the United Kingdom by
Butler & Tanner Ltd
Frome, Somerset, UK

Foreword

Introduction

More than 4 years have passed since the first modern trials of non-myeloablative stem cell transplantation (NST) were reported at the Annual Meeting of the American Society of Hematology in Orlando.[1-3] Since then there has been a steady increase in interest in NST.[4] As viewed today many of the initial regimens explored by Santos and Thomas in the early 1970s would be considered non-ablative or at least of reduced intensity.[5] However, modern NST developed with the recognition that alloreactive donor lymphocytes provided therapeutically as donor lymphocyte infusions (DLI) could mediate a powerful antileukemia effect (particularly in chronic myelogenous leukemia).[6-9]

As currently conceived, NST is being explored as
- a method of harnessing the graft-versus-malignancy (GVM) effect in older and medically debilitated patients
- a safer and less toxic alternative to conventional myeloablative conditioning
- a method of obtaining mixed chimerism with less toxicity in diseases where high dose therapy is unnecessary (e.g. benign disorders) or for tolerance induction.

The role of purine analogs in NST

The introduction of the purine analogs with their potent immunosuppressive activity was also instrumental in the development of NST[10,11] and the vast majority of NST trials have used fludarabine as part of the preparative regimen. The optimal preparative regimens for NST have not been defined, but it is likely that the use of purine analogs will continue to play a major role in their development. The immunosuppressive effects of deoxyadenosine and its analogs have been demonstrated by
- lymphopenia seen after purine analog administration
- prolonged depression of CD4+ and CD8+ lymphocyte counts after purine analog administration
- the occurrence of opportunistic infection
- the occurrence of transfusion associated graft-versus-host disease (GVHD) when non-irradiated white cell transfusions are administered.[12-14]

Although in principle many of these immunosuppressive effects could be considered deleterious, in the context of allogeneic transplantation, they provide a strong rationale to explore these agents further. These immunosuppressive effects could allow engraftment of allogeneic progenitor cells, while also providing antitumor activity against a variety of malignancies, and biochemically modulating the actions of other chemotherapeutic agents thus improving their antitumor efficacy.

Biochemical modulation describes the influence of one drug on the metabolism or actions of a second drug. In the context of NST, these efforts have been directed towards (a) increasing the intracellular dose intensity of ara-C used primarily in the myelogenous leukemias and (b) potentially inhibiting the mechanisms of alkylator-induced DNA repair.[15,16] Ara-C, when it has been phosphorylated to the proximal triphosphate (ara-CTP), is the most efficacious drug in the treatment of myelogenous leukemias. The rate-limiting enzyme in this process is deoxycytidine kinase, an enzyme that is regulated by nucleotide deoxy-CTP. Thus decreasing the levels of dCTP would result in increased production of ara-CTP. dCTP is generated through *de novo* pathways catalyzed by ribonucleotide reductase; *in vitro* studies identified the triphosphate of fludarabine as an effective inhibitor of this enzyme.[16,17] Infusion of fludarabine prior to ara-C therapy potentiated ara-CTP accumulation in blasts, and therefore improved the clinical response. Thus the fludarabine/ara-C and fludarabine/ara-C/granulocyte-colony stimulating factor (G-CSF) (FA and FLAG) regimens were developed at the M. D. Anderson Cancer Center.[18]

The second rationale, which focuses largely on inhibiting mechanisms of DNA repair, developed from the observation that nucleotide analogs must be incorporated into DNA to cause cell death. Activation of DNA repair allows nucleotide analogs to be incorporated into the DNA of quiescent cells. There are many different types of DNA repair:

- repair of DNA damage induced by alkylating agents and interstrand cross-linking requires DNA synthesis
- adduct repair provides an opportunity for incorporation of nucleoside analogs into the DNA of quiescent cells
- incision DNA repair, where deoxynucleotides are removed and then normal deoxynucleotides are added. The most prevalent types are base excision, nucleotide excision, DNA cross-link and mismatch repair.

These are distinct mechanisms of action that call for the replacement of different numbers of nucleotides. For example, base excision repair, which is most closely associated with alkylation of DNA bases, generally only replaces 1–4 nucleotides. Nucleoside excision repair caused by, for example, chlorambucil

Table 1. Response to alkylator therapy, fludarabine monotherapy or fludarabine + cyclophosphamide (FC) in patients with lymphoid malignancies

Prior therapy		Overall response (%CR + PR)		
Alkylators	Fludarabine	Alkylators	Fludarabine	FC
None	None	43	70	85
Resistant	None	< 5	38*	60
Resistant	Resistant	< 5	< 5	38

or UV replaces 27–29 nucleotides (3 turns of the helix). DNA cross-link repair is induced by alkylating agents (cyclophosphamide, melphalan, busulfan, etc.) and allows the incorporation of up to 100 nucleotides.[19] There is therefore an increased probability of incorporating a nucleotide analog into DNA if nuecleoside excision repair or DNA cross-link repair is induced.

Fludarabine interferes with the DNA repair mechanism induced by cyclophosphamide in a schedule-dependent way. Combinations of fludarabine + cyclophosphamide (FC) or fludarabine + platinum + ara-C have been used successfully in the treatment of a number of lymphoid malignancies, including patients refractory to each agent alone (Table 1).[22] Purine analogs may also mediate immunosuppressive activity via dysregulation of or interference in signal transduction.[23,24] This is an area that requires extensive investigation.

The International Workshop on NST

This book was conceived during the First International Workshop of Non-myeloablative Stem Cell Transplantation (iwNST) in St Lucia, West Indies. During two days of intensive discussion more than 40 investigators in the field shared their experience with NST. This book intends to summarize the most relevant information from the meeting and share it with those interested in the field. For us the meeting was a wonderful challenge and the number of new protocols and collaborations it brings will measure its success.

Our hope is that NST will provide new therapeutic strategies for improving the cure rate and quality of life for patients of all ages with malignant and non-malignant disorders. If this assumption proves correct, this may be the first edition of many future textbooks on NST.

Sergio Giralt and Shimon Slavin

References

1. Giralt S, Estey E, van Besien K, Rondón G, O'Brien S, Khouri I, Gajewski J, Mehra R, Claxton D, Beran M, Andersson B, Przepiorka D, Koller C, Korblau S, Albitar M, Körbling M, Kantarjian H, Champlin R. Induction of graft-versus-leukemia without myeloablative therapy using allogeneic PBSC after purine analog containing regimens. *Blood* 1996; 88 (Suppl. 1): 614a.

2. Khouri I, Keating M, Przepiorka D, O'Brien S, Giralt S, Körbling M, Champlin R. Engraftment and induction of GVL with fludarabine based non-ablative preparative regimens in patients with chronic lymphocytic leukemia and lymphoma. *Blood* 1996; 88 (Suppl. 1): 301a.

3. Slavin S, Nagler A, Naperstek E, Ackerstein A, Kapelushnik Y, Varadi G, Kirschbaum M, Ben-Yosef R, Samuel S, Or R. Immunotherapy of leukemia in conjunction with non-myeloablative conditioning: engraftment of blood stem cells and eradication of host leukemia with non-myeloablative conditioning based on fludarabine and anti-thymocyte globulin. *Blood* 1996; 88 (Suppl. 1): 614a

4. Giralt S. Non-myeloablative stem cell transplantation: lessons from the first generation trials. *Leuk Lymphoma Updates* 1999; 2: 4–7.

5. Thomas E, Storb R, Clift R, Fefer A, Johnson L, Neiman PE, Lerner KG, Glucksberg H, Buckner CD. Bone marrow transplantation. *N Engl J Med* 1975; 292: 832–43 & 895–902.

6. Slavin S, Or R, Naparstek E, Ackerstein A, Weiss L. Cellular-mediated immunotherapy of leukemia in conjunction with autologous and allogeneic bone marrow transplantation in experimental animals and man. *Blood* 1988; 72 (Suppl. 1): 407a.

7. Slavin S, Naparstek E, Nagler A, Ackerstein A, Kapelushnik Y, Or R. Allogeneic cell therapy for relapsed leukemia following bone marrow transplantation with donor peripheral blood lymphocytes. *Exp Hematol* 1995; 23: 1553–62.

8. Kolb H, Schattenberg A, Goldman J, Hertenstein B, Jacobsen N, Arcese W, Ljungman P, Ferrant A, Verdonck L, Niederwieser D. Graft-versus-leukemia effect of donor lymphocyte transfusions in marrow grafted patients. *Blood* 1995; 86: 2041–50.

9. Naparstek E, Or R, Nagler A, Cividalli G, Engelhard D, Aker M, Gimon Z, Manny N, Sacks T, Tochner Z, Weiss L, Samuel S, Brautbar C, Hale G, Waldmann H, Steinberg S M, Slavin S. T-cell-depleted allogeneic bone marrow transplantation for acute leukaemia using Campath-1 antibodies and post-transplant administration of donor's peripheral blood lymphocytes for prevention of relapse. *Br J Haematol* 1995; 89: 506–15.

10. Plunkett W, Sanders P. Metabolism and action of purine analogs. *Pharmacol Ther* 1991; 49: 239–45.

11. Champlin R, Khouri I, Komblau S, Molidrem J, Giralt S. Reinventing bone marrow transplantation. Nonmyeloablative preparative regimens and induction of graft-vs-malignancy effect. *Oncology* 1999; 13: 621–8.

12. Keating MJ, O'Brien S, Lerner S, Koller C, Beran M, Robertson LE, Freireich EJ, Estey E, Kantarjian H. Long-term follow-up of patients with chronic lymphocytic leukemia (CLL) receiving fludarabine regimens as initial therapy. *Blood* 1998; 92: 1165–71.

13. Anaissie E, Kontoyiannis DP, Kantarjian H, Elting L, Robertson LE, Keating M. Listeriosis in patients with chronic lymphocytic leukemia who were treated with fludarabine and prednisone. *Ann Intern Med* 1992; 117: 466–9.

14. Williamson LM, Wimperis JZ, Wood ME, Woodcock B. Fludarabine treatment and transfusion-associated graft-versus-host disease. *Lancet* 1996; 348: 472–3.

15. Plunkett W, Heinemann V, Estey E, Keating M. Pharmacologically directed design of leukemia therapy. *Hamatologie Bluttransfusion* 1990; 33: 610–3.

16. Estey E, Plunkett W, Dixon D, Keating M, McCredie K, Freireich EJ. Variables predicting response to high dose cytosine arabinoside therapy in patients with refractory acute leukemia. *Leukemia* 1987; 1: 580–3.

17. Gandhi V, Estey E, Keating M, Plunkett W. Fludarabine potentiates metabolism of cytarabine in patients with acute myelogenous leukemia during therapy. *J Clin Oncol* 1993; 11: 116–24.

18. Estey E, Plunkett W, Gandhi V, Rios M, Kantarjian H, Keating M. Fludarabine and arabinosylcytosine therapy of refractory and relapsed acute myelogenous leukemia. *Leuk Lymphoma* 1993; 9: 343–50.

19. Lindahl T, Wood RD. Quality control by DNA repair. *Science* 1999; 286 1897–905.

20. Li L, Keating MJ, Plunkett W, Yang LY. Fludarabine-mediated repair inhibition of cisplatin-induced DNA lesions in human chronic myelogenous leukemia-blast crisis K562 cells: induction of synergistic cytotoxicity independent of reversal of apoptosis resistance. *Mol Pharmacol* 1997; 52: 798–806.

21. Gandhi V, Huang P, Plunkett W. Fludarabine inhibits DNA replication: a rationale for its use in the treatment of acute leukemias. *Leuk Lymphoma* 1994; 14 (Suppl. 2): 3–9.

22. Keating MJ, O'Brien S, McLaughlin P, Dimopoulos M, Gandhi V, Plunkett W, Lerner S, Kantarjian H, Estey E. Clinical experience with fludarabine in hemato-oncology. *Hematol Cell Ther* 1996; 38 (Suppl. 2): S83–91.

23. Frank DA, Mahajan S, Ritz J. Fludarabine-induced immunosuppression is associated with inhibition of STAT1 signalling. *Nature Med* 1999; 5: 444–7.

24. Genini D, Budihardjo I, Plunkett W, Wang X, Carrera CJ, Cottam HB, Carson DA, Leoni LM. Nucleotide requirements for the *in vitro* activation of the apoptosis protein-activating factor-1-mediated caspase pathway. *J Biol Chem* 2000; 275: 29–34.

Contents

Contributors

J Barrett
National Institute of Health
Building 10, Room 7C 103
9000 Rockville
Bethesda, MD 20892
USA

P Becker
Department Hematology/Oncology
University of Massachusetts
Worcester, MA 01655
USA

K Blume
BMT Program
Stanford University Medical Center
300 Pasteur Drive
Stanford, CA 94305
USA

AM Carella
Coordinator N.O.A Hematology -
Dipartimento di Ematologia
NOA Emataologia ed Autotrapianto
Azienda Ospedale San Martino
Largo Rosanna Benzi, 10
Genoa 16142
Italy

J Carlson
University of Massachusetts Medical Center
NRI Building - Room 211
55 Lake Avenue North
Worcester, MA 01655
USA

R Champlin
Bone Marrow Transplant Unit
University of Texas
M. D. Anderson Cancer Center
1515 Holcombe Boulevard
Houston, TX 77030
USA

TR Chauncey
UW School of Medicine Box 358280
Seattle VA Medical Center
1660 South Columbian Way
Seattle, WA 98108
USA

R Childs
National Institute of Health
NHBL, 10/7C103, 10 Center Drive
Bethesda, MD 20892
USA

GA Colvin
Department Hematology/Oncology
University of Massachusetts
Worcester, MA 01655
USA

M Dooner
University of Massachusetts Medical Center
NRI Building - Room 211
55 Lake Avenue North
Worcester, MA 01655
USA

R Emmons
Department of Hematology/Oncology
University of Massachusetts
Worcester, MA 01655
USA

G Georges
Fred Hutchinson Cancer Research Center
1100 Fairview Avenue North
Seattle, WA 98109
USA

S Giralt
Bone Marrow Transplant Unit
The University of Texas
M. D. Anderson Cancer Center
1515 Holcombe Boulevard
Box 065
Houston, TX 77030
USA

E Goulmy
Leiden University Medical Centre
Building One, E3-Q
PO Box 9600
Leiden 2300 RC
Netherlands

C Hsieh
University of Massachusetts Medical Center
NRI Building - Room 211
55 Lake Avenue North
Worcester, MA 01655
USA

IF Khouri
Bone Marrow Transplant Unit
The University of Texas
M. D. Anderson Cancer Center
1515 Holcombe Blvd
Box 65
Houston, TX 77030
USA

JF Lambert
University of Massachusetts Medical Center
NRI Building - Room 211
55 Lake Avenue North
Worcester, MA 01655
USA

DG Maloney
Fred Hutchinson Cancer Research Center
1100 Fairview Avenue, North
Seattle, WA 98109
USA

M Maris
Fred Hutchinson Cancer Research Center
1100 Fairview Avenue North
Seattle, WA 98109
USA

C McAuliffe
University of Massachusetts Medical Center
NRI Building - Room 211
55 Lake Avenue North
Worcester, MA 01655
USA

P McSweeney
Bone Marrow Transplant Program
University of Colorado
4200 East Ninth Ave
Box B190
Denver, CO 80262
USA

C Miller
University of Massachusetts Medical Center
NRI Building - Room 211
55 Lake Avenue North
Worcester, MA 01655
USA

A Molina
City of Hope National Medical Center
1500 E Duarte Road
Duarte, CA 91010
USA

A Nagler
Bone Marrow Transplantation Department
Hadassah University Hospital
PO Box 12000
Jerusalem 91120
Israel

D Niederwieser
Department of Haematology
University of Leipzig
Leipzig
Germany

R Or
Department of Bone Marrow Transplantation
Hadassah University Hospital
PO Box 12000
Jerusalem 91120
Israel

PJ Quesenberry
Two Biotech
373 Plantation Street, Suite 3202
Worcester, MA 01605
USA

J Reilly
University of Massachusetts Medical Center
NRI Building - Room 211
55 Lake Avenue North
Worcester, MA 01655
USA

BM Sandmaier
Clinical Research Division
Fred Hutchinson Cancer Research Center
1100 Fairview Avenue North
Seattle, WA 98109
USA

JA Shizuru
Stanford SHS H1353
USA

S Slavin
Department of Bone Marrow Transplantation
and Cancer Immunotherapy
Hadassah University Hospital
PO Box 12000
Jerusalem 91120
Israel

FM Stewart
Department Hematology/Oncology
University of Massachusetts
Worcester, MA 01655
USA

R Storb
Clincial Research Division
Fred Hutchinson Cancer Research Ctr
1100 Fairview Avenue North
Seattle, WA 98109
USA

M Sykes
Harvard Medical School
Transplantation Biology Research Center
Massachusetts General Hospital
MGH East, Bldg149-5102, 13th Street
Boston, MA 02129
USA

H Wang
University Massachusetts Medical School
55 Lake Avenue North
Worcester, MA 01655
USA

K Werne
University of Massachusetts Medical Center
NRI Building - Room 211
55 Lake Avenue North
Worcester, MA 01655
USA

A Woolfrey
Fred Hutchinson Cancer Research Center
1100 Fairveiw Avenue North
Seattle, WA 98109
USA

JM Zaucha
Fred Hutchinson Cancer Research Center
1100 Fairview Avenue North
Seattle, WA 980109
USA

S Zhong
University of Massachusetts Medical Center
NRI Building - Room 211
55 Lake Avenue North
Worcester, MA 01655
USA

New frontiers in cancer therapy

Non-myeloablative stem cell transplantation (NST)

Section 1 – Preclinical studies

Maternal–fetal natural mixed chimerism and bilateral transplantation tolerance

S Slavin

B one marrow transplantation (BMT) is an important clinical tool for treating patients with a wide variety of malignant and non-malignant diseases. Unfortunately, BMT is hazardous, expensive and associated with high rates of procedure-related morbidity and mortality. As will be discussed below, we have reason to believe that safer and less costly BMT procedures may become available in the near future. Our optimism results from the fact that transplantation tolerance to donor stem cells, which seems to be the key element for successful and safe BMT, can be induced with minimal conditioning based on immunoregulation rather than myeloablation.

Indications for BMT

There are many accepted indications for transplantation of bone marrow-derived stem cells, and the number of indications is continually increasing. Some of the major indications for BMT for both malignant and non-malignant diseases and the rationales for choosing these indications are shown in Table 1.

BMT is associated with high rates of procedure-related toxicity and mortality as well as unavoidable late complications that are frequently caused directly or indirectly by the intensive conditioning administered during the pre-transplant period. Therefore, it would a major advantage if a safer BMT procedure could be introduced using well-tolerated conditioning. Patients with high-risk hematologic malignancies in particular could benefit from a curative procedure at an early stage of the disease, thus avoiding the need for long-term chemotherapy with all the associated complications. Patients with genetic diseases would also benefit at an early stage of their disease, when the chance for complete cure may be much higher.

Transplantation tolerance with no myeloablation

Transplantation tolerance across major histocompatibility complex (MHC) occurs spontaneously in nature, as evidenced by the fact that pregnant females do not reject their conceptus. In fact, as shown by Owens in the 1940s, placen-

Table 1. Common indications for allogeneic stem cell transplantation for life-threatening malignant and non-malignant diseases

- Replacement therapy for diseases caused by deficiency of stem cells (e.g. severe aplastic anemia) or abnormal stem cells (e.g. severe combined immune deficiency)

- Replacement therapy for diseases caused by deficiency of stem cell products (e.g. enzyme deficiency diseases such as Gaucher's disease)

- Replacement of host with donor stem cells in genetic disorders and diseases caused by abnormal stem cells or stem cell progeny (e.g. beta-thalassemia major)

- Replacement of host with donor immuno-hematopoietic cells in malignant hematologic diseases following eradication of tumor cells of host origin with high dose chemoradiotherapy

- Stem cell transplantation for induction of transplantation tolerance as a platform for allogeneic cell therapy with naïve or specific immune donor lymphocytes

- Elimination of self-reactive lymphocytes in conjunction with autologous stem cell transplantation, or replacement of host with donor stem cells in conjunction with allogeneic BMT for the treatment of life-threatening autoimmune diseases

- Stem cell transplantation for induction of transplantation tolerance to donor organ allografts and xenografts

tal parabiosis *in utero* leads to permanent mixed chimerism and bilateral transplantation tolerance.[1] These observations led to an experiment by Billingham *et al.* that showed that infusion of parental stem cells into neonates with no exogenous immunosuppressive treatment resulted in mixed chimerism and permanent transplantation tolerance to donor alloantigens.[2] This suggested that there is a window of opportunity, shortly after delivery, during which tolerance can be induced without the need for conditioning. Tolerant recipients were shown to be chimeras with only a small proportion of donor cells. However, without corroborating evidence that transplantation tolerance could be intentionally induced, the approach could not be applied in clinical practice for immunocompetent recipients. Nonetheless, these experiments suggested that stable mixed chimerism is feasible and may be responsible for successful induction of transplantation tolerance to donor alloantigens. In addition, these observations indicated that if antigen specific unresponsiveness can be achieved with no myeloablative immunosuppression, it should be possible to accomplish the same goal with minimal or no conditioning, by immune regulation rather than immunosuppression, analogous to the mechanism of unresponsiveness which operates at the stage of 'self/non-self' discrimination and during pregnancy. Since transplantation tolerance is induced by engraftment of stem cells, development of mixed chimerism may be the only critical requirement for induction of host-versus-graft (HVG) and graft-versus-host (GVH) unresponsiveness. Thus non-myeloablative stem cell transplantation (NST) resulting in mixed chimerism, rather than full donor chimerism, may be the safest method for transplanting donor stem cells.

Starting in 1976, we published a series of papers addressing the feasibility of establishing transplantation tolerance and bilateral tolerance by mixed chimerism in immunologically mature recipients across MHC.[3–8] Experiments in mice,[3–5] rats[6] and dogs[7] showed that following non-myeloablative conditioning with well tolerated total lymphoid irradiation (TLI), recipients experienced durable engraftment of donor bone marrow and skin or perfused organ allografts, with no graft-versus-host disease (GVHD). In mixed chimeras, HVG and GVH were neutralized simultaneously without the need for any post-transplant immunosuppression. However, the mechanisms responsible for the balanced equilibrium in mixed chimeras were not understood.[9] After TLI, circulating and tissue-bound T cells were eliminated[4] and newly formed T cells acquired tolerance to protein antigens[10] and alloantigens.[3–8] Circulating and spleen cells analyzed by FACS before new T cells were detectable, were large cells carrying the null phenotype.[11] When T cells reappeared the large cell subpopulation decreased, suggesting that the latter played some role in the development of the unresponsive state. These large cells were enriched with hematopoietic progenitor cells,[12] indicating that, upon maturation in the thymus, any new antigen encountered would be regarded as 'self', resulting in apoptosis of self-reactive T cells. Following TLI, enrichment with such immature cells enabled the recipients to develop tolerance, mainly as a result of clonal deletion.[13] Following non-myeloablative conditioning, between the time when no mature T cells are present and the appearance of uncommitted immature cells, allografts or any protein antigen will be regarded as self.

Spleen cells from recipient chimeric mice with intact skin allografts did not cause GVHD and could transfer their specific tolerance to skin allografts in secondary recipients.[14] Tolerant chimeras had large mononuclear 'null' cells (negative for Thy1, CD4, CD8 and Ig) that suppressed 100% MLR.[15] Suppressor cells of MLR were soybean agglutinin positive large cells that looked like stem cells, and had suppressive functions that were identical to those of normal marrow cells. Interestingly, although suppressor cells were present in chimeras, specific unresponsiveness could best be explained by clonal deletion and anergy of residual cells.[13,14]

Ildstad and Sachs[16] and subsequently Sykes and Sachs[17–19] showed similar results, except that they used TBI and infused two sets of cells rather than protecting the mouse's own cells and infusing allogeneic lymphocytes. The former studies were continued by Starzl et al.,[20] who showed that donor cells could not be detected in non-rejector mice using PCR analysis, implying that even micro-chimerism may enhance graft acceptance and donor tolerance induction. More recently, based on an improved understanding of the mechanism of alloimmune responses and the ability to block the immune response by suppressing co-stimulation, transplantation tolerance has been induced using truly minimal conditioning.[21] We reasoned that if clonal deletion could not be accomplished by mimicking natural central tolerance induction, there may be other ways to induce donor specific clonal deletion.[22] In clinical BMT, there are two ways to achieve engraftment without GVHD

- complete T-cell depletion in both the graft and the host, leading to no GVHD and no rejection, but this requires aggressive hazardous conditioning
- or balancing the T cells in the graft and the host to down regulate host antidonor and donor antihost alloreactive T cells by a mechanism of veto.[9]

However, the optimal way to achieve engraftment without GVHD would be to deplete only the relevant T cells in the graft and host, thus inducing apoptosis/cytoreduction of both host-reactive T cells to prevent GVHD and donor-reactive T cells to prevent rejection, respectively.

Studies have shown that reduced intensity conditioning can be very useful in conjunction with clonal deletion[9,22] or immunoregulation by costimulation blockade.[21] The more effective the conditioning, the better the tolerance induction, with fewer donor cells needed for durable engraftment of donor hematopoietic cells, especially following non-myeloablative conditioning. In contrast, the more intensive the pre-grafting immunosuppression, the more aggressive the GVHD, suggesting some possible down-regulation between host and donor immunohematopoietic cells. Engraftment could be facilitated by donor T cells, hence, when using T-cell depleted stem cell allografts to completely prevent GVHD, higher numbers of donor stem cells were required in both mice[24] and man.[25] In summary, mildly immunosuppressed hosts required either higher numbers of donor stem cells or induction of donor-specific clonal deletion. These results suggested that immunosuppression could be achieved without myeloablation in the clinic and that a window of immunosuppression would prevent rejection of donor stem cells required to induce transplantation tolerance.

In future, treatments based on immunoregulation rather than non-discriminatory elimination of alloreactive cells in the recipient should render patients less prone to infectious complications and secondary cancer. Examples of tolerance induction to autologous or allogeneic lymphocytes, respectively, without exogenous immunosuppression include:

- spontaneous induction of self-tolerance induced by deletion of self-reactive T cells in the thymus
- peripheral antigen-dependent anergy that down-regulates potentially self-reactive T cells that may escape central clonal deletion in the thymus
- immune recovery of recipients of mismatched bone marrow allografts following T cell depleted stem cell transplantation with no GVHD.

Based on experimental data and cumulative clinical experience it can be concluded that donor alloreactive T cells are most dangerous following intensive conditioning, which includes a combination of immunosuppression and myeloablation. In addition to the degree of mismatching, which determines the alloreactive potential of immunocompetent donor lymphocytes, the intensity of GVHD is also directly proportional to the intensity of the conditioning. Hence, following intensive myeloablative conditioning, control of GVHD may require one of the following approaches:

- T-cell depletion (preferred in mismatched donor–recipient pairs) to control GVHD while avoiding post-transplant immunosuppression
- use of non-alloreactive donor T cells for immunological reconstruction and safe adoptive transfer of donor immunity while preventing or minimizing GVHD.

Following non-myeloablative conditioning, donor T cells can facilitate donor stem cell engraftment with an acceptable risk of GVHD, depending on the intensity of the conditioning, since mixed chimerism may partially protect the host from GVHD. Hence, following NST, when residual T cells of host origin need to be controlled, the role of donor T cells in facilitation of engraftment is much more critical. Accordingly, alloreactive T cells may play an important role in graft facilitation. Under such circumstances, the following can be anticipated:

- T-cell depleted allografts may be highly susceptible to rejection by residual host T cells
- non-alloreactive T cells cannot facilitate engraftment because of the continuous presence of residual alloreactive host T cells.

An inverse relationship exists between the stem cell dose given and the degree of specific HVG unresponsiveness. At a low frequency of cytotoxic

Table 2. Positive and negative aspects of immunocompetent T cells in BMT

Positive aspects

* Protection against infectious complications

* Induction of unresponsiveness[26]

* Down-regulation by host T cells of donor T cells and control of GVHD[27]

* Down-regulation by donor T cells of host T cells, control of graft rejection and facilitation of engraftment[24,25]

* Reaction against host hematopoietic cells (malignant, genetically abnormal or self-reactive) by donor cells eliciting a graft-versus-malignancy, graft-versus-genetically abnormal stem cells or graft-versus-autoimmunity effect[28–35]

Negative aspects

* T cells are the major obstacles to successful transplantation of bone marrow and organ allografts: host T cells cause rejection and donor T cells mediate both acute and chronic GVHD.

T-lymphocyte precursor cells (CTLp) very few cells will engraft. At a high percentage of CTLp cells the chance of achieving mixed chimerism is low, instead full donor chimerism is more likely (for more details see Chapter 3). The positive and negative roles played by alloreactive T cells in BMT are summarized in Table 2.

In summary

Experimental and clinical application of different treatments to control the immune system, concentrating on minimal conditioning to accomplish bilateral transplantation tolerance of HVG and GVH responses is the main focus of interest. The goal is to take advantage of immune regulation as a basis for safe and well-tolerated allogeneic stem cell transplantation to be followed by cell therapy. Better approaches for the treatment of malignant and non-malignant diseases, using immune cells to eliminate, replace or control malignant and non-malignant cells will hopefully be developed.

Acknowledgements

We would like to thank the following for their ongoing support: Baxter International Corporation; Max & Adi Moss Research Laboratory; Ryna & Melvin Cohen; The Szydlowsky Foundation; Donald & Ronne Hess and Joanne & David Morrison; The Gabriella Rich Foundation; The Himmelfarb Foundation. The work was carried out at The Danny Cunniff Leukemia Research Laboratory.

References

1.   Owen RD. Immunogenetic consequences of vascular anastomoses between bovine twins. *Science* 1945; 102: 400.

2.   Billingham RE, Brent L, Medavar PB. Actively acquired tolerance to foreign cells. *Nature* 1953; 172: 606.

3.   Slavin S, Strober S, Fuks Z, Kaplan HS. Long-term survival of skin allografts in mice treated with fractionated total lymphoid irradiation. *Science* 1976; 193: 1252–4.

4.   Slavin S, Strober S, Fuks Z, Kaplan HS. Induction of specific tissue transplantation tolerance using fractionated total lymphoid irradiation in adult mice: long-term survival of allogeneic bone marrow and skin grafts. *J Exp Med* 1977; 146: 34–48.

5.   Slavin S, Fuks Z, Kaplan HS, Strober S. Transplantation of allogeneic bone marrow without graft vs host disease using total lymphoid irradiation. *J Exp Med* 1978; 147: 963–72.

6.   Slavin S, Reitz B, Bieber CP, Kaplan HS, Strober S. Transplantation tolerance in adult rats using total lymphoid irradiation (TLI): Permanent survival of skin, heart and marrow allografts. *J Exp Med* 1978; 147: 700–07.

7.   Howard RJ, Sutherland DER, Lum CT, Lewis WI, Kim TH, Slavin S, Najarian JS. Kidney allograft survival in dogs treated with total lymphoid irradiation. *Ann Surg* 1981; 193: 196–200.

8.   Slavin S. Total lymphoid irradiation. *Immunol Today* 1987; 3: 88.

9.   Prigozhina T, Gurevitch O, Slavin S. Non-myeloablative conditioning to induce bilateral tolerance after allogeneic bone marrow transplantation in mice. *Exp Hematol* 1999; 27: 1503–10.

10. Zan-Bar I, Slavin S, Strober S. Induction and mechanism of tolerance to bovine serum albumin after total lymphoid irradiation (TLI). *J Immunol* 1978; 121: 1400–04.

11. Weigensberg M, Morecki S, Weiss L, Fuks Z, Slavin S. Suppression of cell mediated immune responses following total lymphoid irradiation (TLI). 1. Characterization of suppressor cell of the mixed lymphocyte reaction. *J Immunol* 1984; 132: 971–8.

12. Slavin S, Seidel HJ. Hematopoietic activity in bone marrow chimeras prepared with total lymphoid irradiation (TLI). *Exp Hematol* 1982; 10: 206–16.

13. Morecki S, Leshem B, Weigensberg M, Bar S, Slavin S. Functional clonal deletion versus active suppression in transplantation tolerance induced by total lymphoid irradiation (TLI). *Transplantation* 1985; 40: 201–10.

14. Morecki S, Leshem B, Eid A, Slavin S. Alloantigen persistence in induction and maintenance of transplantation tolerance. *J Exp Med* 1987; 165: 1468–80.

15. Slavin S, Strober S. Induction of allograft tolerance after total lymphoid irradiation (TLI): Development of suppressor cells of the mixed leukocyte reaction MLR. *J Immunol* 1979; 123: 942–6.

16. Ildstad ST, Sachs DH. Reconstitution with syngeneic plus allogeneic or xenogeneic bone marrow leads to specific acceptance of allografts or xenografts. *Nature* 1984; 307: 168–70.

17. Sykes M, Chester CH, Sachs DH. Protection from graft-vs-host disease in fully allogeneic chimeras by prior administration of T cell-depleted syngeneic bone marrow. *Transplantation* 1988; 46: 327–30.

18. Sykes M, Sachs DH. Mixed allogeneic chimerism as an approach to transplantation tolerance. *Immunol Today* 1988; 9: 23–27.

19. Sykes M, Sachs DH. Bone marrow transplantation as a means of inducing tolerance. *Semin Immunol* 1990; 2: 401–17.

20. Starzl TE, Demetris AJ, Murase N, Trucco M, Thomson AW, Rao AS. The lost chord: microchimerism and allograft survival. *Immunol Today* 1996; 12: 577–84.

21. Werkerle T, Kurtz J, Ito H, Ronquillo JV, Dong V, Zhao G, Shaffer J, Sayegh MH, Sykes M. Allogeneic bone marrow transplantation with co-stimulatory blockade induces macrochimerism and tolerance without cytoreductive host treatment. *Nat Med* 2000; 4: 464–9.

22. Prigozhina T, Gurevitch O, Zhu J, Slavin S. Permanent and specific transplantation tolerance induced by a non-myeloablative treatment to a wide variety of allogeneic tissues. *Transplantation* 1997; 63: 1394–9.

23. Storb R, Yu C, Barnett T, Wagner JL, Deeg HJ, Nash RA, Kiem HP, McSweeney P, Seidel K, Georges G, Zaucha JM. Stable mixed hematopoietic chimerism in dog leukocyte antigen-identical littermate dogs given lymph node irradiation before and pharmacological immunosuppression after marrow transplantation. *Blood* 1999; 94: 1131–6.

24. Bachar-Lustig E, Rachamim N, Li HW, Lan F, Reisner Y. Megadose of T cell-depleted bone marrow overcomes MHC barriers in sublethally irradiated mice. *Nat Med* 1995; 1: 1268–73.

25. Reisner Y, Martelli MF. Bone marrow transplantation across HLA barriers by increasing the number of transplanted cells. *Immunol Today* 1995; 16: 437–40.

26. Waldmann H, Cobbold S. How do monoclonal antibodies induce tolerance? A role for infectious tolerance? *Ann Rev Immunol* 1998; 16: 619–44.

27. Weiss L, Slavin S. Prevention and treatment of graft vs host disease by down-regulation of anti-host reactivity with veto cells of host origin. *Bone Marrow Transplant* 1999; 23: 1139–43.

28. Slavin S, Naparstek E, Nagler A, Ackerstein A, Samuel S, Kapelushnik J, Brautbar C, Or R. Allogeneic cell therapy with donor peripheral blood cells and recombinant human interleukin-2 to treat leukemia relapse post allogeneic bone marrow transplantation. *Blood* 1996; 87: 2195–204.

29. van Besien K, Sobocinski KA, Rowlings PA, Murphy SC, Armitage JO, Bishop MR, Chaekal OK, Gale RP, Klein JP, Lazarus HM, McCarthy PL Jr, Raemaekers JM, Reiffers J, Phillips GL, Schattenberg AV, Verdonck LF, Vose JM, Horowitz MM. Allogeneic bone marrow transplantation for low-grade lymphoma. *Blood* 1998; 92: 1832–6.

30. Or R, Mehta J, Naparstek E, Okon E, Cividalli G, Slavin S. Successful T cell-depleted allogeneic bone marrow transplantation in a child with recurrent multiple extramedullary plasmacytomas. *Bone Marrow Transplant* 1992; 10: 381–2.

31. Tricot G, Vesole DH, Jagannath S, Hilton J, Munshi N, Barlogie B. Graft-versus-myeloma effect: Proof of principle. *Blood* 1996; 87: 1196–8.

32. Eibl B, Schwaighofer H, Nachbaur D, Marth C, Gächter A, Knapp R, Böck G, Gassner C, Schiller L, Petersen F, Niederwieser D. Evidence for a graft-versus-tumor effect in a patient treated with marrow ablative chemotherapy and allogeneic bone marrow transplantation for breast cancer. *Blood* 1996, 88: 1501–08.

33. Childs RW, Clave E, Tisdale J, Plante M, Hensel N, Barrett J. Successful treatment of metastatic renal cell carcinoma with a nonmyeloablative allogeneic peripheral-blood progenitor-cell transplant: evidence for a graft-versus-tumor effect. *J Clin Oncol* 1999; 17: 2044–4.

34. Kapelushnik J, Or R, Aker M, Cividalli G, Nagler A, Naparstek E, Varadi G, Ackerstein A, Amar A, Slavin S. Allogeneic cell therapy of severe beta thalassemia major by displacement of host stem cells in mixed chimera by donor blood lymphocytes. *Bone Marrow Transplant* 1996; 19: 96–8.

35. Slavin S, Nagler A, Naparstek E, Varadi G, Ben-Yosef R, Or R. Graft vs autoimmune lymphocytes (GVA) following allogeneic bone marrow transplantation in a patient with chronic myelogenous leukemia and severe systemic psoriasis and psoriatic polyarthritis. *Exp Hematol,* in press.

Stem cell transplantation without myeloablation in immunocompetent recipients

PJ Quesenberry, FM Stewart, P Becker, R Emmons,
C Hsieh, K Werme, H Habibian, J Reilly, C McAuliffe,
M Dooner, J Carlson, C Miller, JF Lambert, GA Colvin,
L Pang, BO Benoit, S Zhong, H Wang, J Damon

A longstanding dogma has held that the transplantation of bone marrow stem cells into the marrow cavity of animals or humans necessitated treatment that would open space to allow for the seeding of marrow stem cells. This dogma persists to the present day, although a substantial amount of information is now available indicating that stem cell competition, rather than space, is the primary determinant of stem cell engraftment in the transplant setting where immune barriers do not exist (i.e. syngeneic or autologous transplantation). Our own studies, following on the work of Brecher and colleagues[1] and consistent with published work by several other groups,[2-5] attempted to engraft 200 million male BALB/c cells into non-treated female BABL/c hosts, tracking male DNA in the organs of the transplanted female BALB/c mice.[6] Up to 40 million cells were given intravenously for five consecutive days and engraftment was evaluated over a 2-year period post-cell infusion. Male DNA was tracked using the PY2 probe for repetitive sequences on the Y chromosome, and detected either by Southern blot analysis or fluorescent in situ hybridization (FISH) with a Y painting probe. These studies showed extraordinarily high levels of engraftment in marrow after several years. These levels of engraftment were frequently mirrored in spleen, thymus and blood, although sometimes the levels were lower in these organs. In studies in which 50 million marrow cells were given for either one, two, three, four or five injections, the observed engraftment was very close to the maximum theoretically predicted engraftment, assuming a total mouse cellularity of 300 million cells, and further assuming that the number of differentiated cells represents the stem cell number.[7] In a similar fashion, graded doses of marrow cells were given using a 5-day schedule, with the same conclusion. When individual animals were analyzed in these engraftment studies, some showed up to twice the expected level of engraftment.[7] These data suggest that there was almost quantitative engraftment at the stem cell level in the non-myeloablated host. This is consistent with the concept that stem cell competition is the main (if not the only) determinant of engraftment in stem cell transplants where immune barriers are not operative. Work by Hendrix and colleagues[8] evaluating immediate homing of purified stem cells also arrived at the conclusion that stem cell homing was not augmented by myeloablative therapy, but instead was modestly diminished.

The engrafting stem cells were non-cycling, as determined by *in vitro* thymidine suicide or *in vivo* hydroxyurea techniques.[9] The actual cycle status of the most primitive stem cell as represented by the lineage negative rhodamine[low] Hoechst[low] (rho[lo] Ho[lo]) cell remains an area of controversy. Bradford and colleagues,[10] using continuous oral bromodeoxyuridine (BRDU) administration, reported that the majority of lineage negative rho[lo] Ho[lo] cells are actually slowly going through cell cycle. The possibility exists, however, that the BRDU incorporation could represent DNA damage and repair, rather than proliferation. Studies addressing this point in our laboratory unfortunately have been inconclusive. However, it is clear that the lineage negative rho[lo] Ho[lo] cell is easily induced into cycle either by *in vitro* exposure to various cytokines, or shortly after *in vivo* engraftment.[11-13] Using an *in vivo* hydroxyurea suicide technique, we showed that approximately half of the engrafting stem cells had entered cell cycle 12 hours post-cell infusion.[13] The engrafting stem cells also moved rapidly to the endosteal surface, where they persisted and then gave rise to osteocytes.[14,15] Purified lineage negative rho[lo] Ho[lo] stem cells effectively engraft in non-myeloablated hosts, however, the engraftment capacity of purified stem cells is much less than that in the original marrow population from which the cells were purified. This suggests either a loss of stem cells in the separation procedures or the existence of syngeneic facilitator cells.[14] This latter possibility has not been supported by preliminary experiments in our laboratory.

Using lineage-negative, Sca-positive, murine-purified stem cells labeled with CFSE, a fluorescent cytoplasmic label, we were able to show that there was a plateau of engraftment at approximately 3 hours. Characteristics of stem cell engraftment into non-myeloablated syngeneic mice are summarized in Table 1.

Table 1. Engraftment in non-myeloablated hosts

1. The engrafting stem cell is quiescent, but is rapidly induced into cell cycle after engraftment
2. The stem cell rapidly moves to the endosteum and persists there
3. Purified lineage rho[lo] Ho[lo] stem cells engraft
4. Infusion of marrow cells gives rise to long-term multi-lineage, multi-organ engraftment
5. Engraftment is determined by stem cell competition

Engraftment in the minimally treated syngeneic host

The hypothesis that syngeneic engraftment is determined solely by stem cell competition suggests that if host stem cells were reduced, the percentage donor chimerism would increase. A number of cytotoxic agents or radiation have the capacity to damage bone marrow stem cells. One of the best studied is whole body irradiation. A large number of previous studies using a variety of stem cell or progenitor assays with or without cytokine stimulation have indicated that D^o values, the value to reduce stem progenitor cells to two thirds of the normal level, range from 40 to 275 centigrade.[16–20] Levels of radiation in the range of 50–150 cGy have relatively modest effects on differentiated hematopoiesis, but are still stem cell toxic. Our own data showed that 100 cGy causes relatively mild and short term (two weeks) depression of platelets and white cells, while having profound and long-lasting effects on the levels of long term engrafting stem cells;[21] levels were reduced to approximately 10% of control. Thus, 100 cGy host irradiation provided a potential treatment that was relatively non-myelotoxic, but stem cell toxic. If stem cell competition is the basis for syngeneic chimerism, then such an approach should increase donor chimerism with minimal toxicity. Infusion of 40 million marrow cells into hosts treated with 100 cGy gave very high levels of chimerism, usually in the range of 60–80%, out to eight months post-cell infusion. Reducing the total cell dose to 10 million cells still resulted in 30–40% chimerism. These data provided an intriguing model for establishing high levels of chimerism in autologous or syngeneic transplantation. This approach could also be potentially useful in various gene therapy settings, however, to be more broadly applicable it would need to be applied to allogeneic transplantation.

Accordingly, we evaluated an H2 mismatched model, B6.SJL, to BALB/c transplantation. Initially, we evaluated BALB/c mice given 100 cGy and infused with 40 million B6.SJL marrow cells – chimerism was not seen. The irradiation doses had to be increased to 400–500 cGy to obtain chimerism. Thus additional tolerization was needed to obtain allochimerism with minimal nontoxic host treatment. One of the approaches we took involved presenting antigen in the presence of costimulator blockade. We used B6.SJL spleen cells for antigen exposure and then blocked the CD40/CD40 ligand costimulator pathway. Ten million B6.SJL spleen cells were given intravenously 10 days prior to transplant. CD40 antibody ligand was given shortly before the spleen cells were administered, and subsequently on days –7, –3, 0 and +3. On day 0 host animals received 100 cGy and were infused with 40 million B6.SJL marrow cells. This resulted in stable, long term chimerism at levels of 30–40% lasting out to over one year post-engraftment. So far, no animal has rejected the graft and there has been no graft-versus-host disease. In addition, at 44 weeks a

Table 2. Allochimeric transplant model

Feature	Mechanism
Minimal host treatment (100 cGy)	Avoids cytokine storm
High levels of stem cells	Inherently tolerizing
Antigen pre-exposure and CD40 ligand antibody blockade	Induces tolerance

small number of engrafted animals accepted a B6.SJL skin graft, but rejected third party grafts, demonstrating that there was specific tolerance to skin grafting. In this model, increasing the cell dose or the antibody dose increased the degree of chimerism. Thus, this is potentially a valuable model for the non-toxic creation of allochimerism that might be applied clinically. Critical features of this allochimeric model are listed in Table 2.

Further characteristics of the engrafting stem cells

Stem cells engrafting in these models were found to have extraordinarily rapid motility. In the presence of various cytokines, particularly stroma-derived factor-one and steel factor, they were also able to extend pseudopods, termed proteopods, which appeared to provide a mechanism for movement and homing. As noted above, these cells were rapidly induced into cell cycle, and it was determined that at various points in the cycle the cells showed marked fluctuation between high and low levels of engraftability. Initial studies showed a loss of engraftment in late S/early G2 phase, and a return of engraftability in the next G1 phase.[22] These marked fluctuations of engraftment appear to relate to the ability of these cells to home, in that at 48 hours post-cytokine exposure (IL-3, IL-6, IL-11 and steel factor), a time when engraftment is markedly impaired, stem cell homing is also impaired. Studies on adhesion proteins revealed a potential mechanism for these fluctuations. It was determined that fluctuations of alpha 4, 5, 6, L-selectin and PECAM-1 correlated with engraftability; these entities being lost or diminished at times of poor engraftability.[23] Lastly, another characteristic of stem cells which is important to consider with regard to interpreting various experimental results is that engraftability shows clear and fairly dramatic circadian rhythms.

References

1. Brecher, G, Ansell JD, Micklem HS, Tjio JH, Cronkite EP. Special proliferative sites are not needed for seeding and proliferation of transfused bone marrow cells in normal syngeneic mice. *PNAS* 1982; 79: 5085–7.

2. Micklem HS, Clarke CM, Evans EP, Ford CE. Fate of chromosome-marked mouse bone marrow cells transfused into normal syngeneic recipients. *Transplantation* 1968; 6: 299–302.

3. Takada A, Takada Y, Ambrus JL. Proliferation of donor spleen and marrow cells in the spleens and bone marrows of unirradiated and irradiated adult mice. *Proc Soc Exp Biol Med* 1970; 136: 222–6.

4. Takada Y, Takada A. Proliferation of donor hematopoietic cells in irradiated and unirradiated host mice. *Transplantation* 1971; 12: 334–8.

5. Saxe DF, Boggs SS, Boggs DR. Transplantation of chromosomally marked syngeneic marrow cells into mice not subjected to hematopoietic stem cell depletion. *Exp Hematol* 1984; 12: 277–83.

6. Stewart FM, Crittenden R, Lowry PA, Pearson-White S, Quesenberry PJ. Long-term engraftment of normal and post-5-fluorouracil murine marrow into normal nonmyeloablated mice. *Blood* 1993; 81: 2566–71.

7. Rao SS, Peters SO, Critten RB, Stewart FM, Ramshaw HS, Quesenberry PJ. Stem cell transplantation in the normal non-myeloablated host: Relationship between cell dose, schedule and engraftment. *Exp Hematol* 1997; 25: 114–21.

8. Hendrikx PJ, Martens ACM, Hagenbeek A, Keij JF, Visser JW. Homing of fluorescently labeled hematopoietic stem cells. *Exp Hematol* 1996; 24: 129–40.

9. Ramshaw HS, Rao SS, Crittenden RB, Peters SO, Weier HU, Quesenberry PJ. Engraftment of bone marrow cells into normal unprepared hosts: Effects of 5-fluorouracil and cell cycle status. *Blood* 1995; 86: 924–9.

10. Bradford GB, Williams B, Rossi R, Bertonello I. Quiescence, cycling and turnover in the primitive hematopoietic stem cell compartment. *Exp Hematol* 1997; 25: 445–53.

11. Peters SO, Kittler EL, Ramshaw HS, Quesenberry PJ. Murine marrow cells expanded in culture with IL-3, IL-6, IL-11, and SCF acquire an engraftment defect in normal hosts. *Exp Hematol* 1995; 23: 461–9.

12. Peters SO, Kittler ELW, Ramshaw HS, Quesenberry PJ. *Ex vivo* expansion of murine marrow cells with interleukin-3, interleukin-6, interleukin-11, and stem cell factor leads to impaired engraftment in irradiated hosts. *Blood* 1996; 87: 30–7.

13. Nilsson SK, Dooner MS, Quesenberry PJ. Synchronized cell-cycle induction of engrafting long-term repopulating stem cells. *Blood* 1997; 90: 4646–50.

14. Nilsson S, Dooner M, Tiarks C, Heinz-Ulrich W, Quesenberry PJ. Potential and distribution of transplanted hematopoietic stem cells in a non-ablated mouse model. *Blood* 1997; 89: 4013–20.

15. Nilsson SK, Dooner MS, Weier HU, Frenkel B, Lian JB, Stein GS, Quesenberry PJ. Cells capable of bone production engraft from whole bone marrow transplants in nonablated mice. *J Exp Med* 1999; 189: 729–34.

16. Kyoizumi S, McCune JM, Namikawa R. Direct evaluation of radiation damage in human hematopoietic progenitor cells *in vitro*. *Radiat Res* 1994; 137: 76–83.

17. Goff JP, Shields DS, Boggs SS, Greenberger JS. Effects of recombinant cytokines on colony formation by irradiated human cord blood CD34+ hematopoietic progenitor cells. *Radiat Res* 1997; 147: 61–9.

18. Trishking AL, Konopliannikov AG. [The radiosensitivity of hematopoietic stem cells from mice forming splenic colonies after 8 and 12 days following bone marrow cell transplantation (CFU-S-8 and CFU-S-12).] *Radiobiologiia* 1992; 32: 207–10.

19. Inoue T, Hirabayashi Y, Mitsui H, Sasaki H, Cronkite EP, Bollis JE, Jr, Bond VP, Yoshida K. Survival of spleen colony forming units (CFU-5) of irradiated bone marrow cells in mice: Evidence for the existence of a radioresistant subfraction. *Exp Hematol* 1995; 23: 1296–300.

20. Scheding S, Media JE, KuKuruga MA, Nakeff A. *In situ* radiation sensitivity of recombinant human granulocyte colony-stimulating factor recruited murine circulating blood and bone marrow progenitor colony-forming unit (CFU) – granulocyte-macrophage and CFU-megakaryocyte: Evidence for possible biologic differences between mobilized blood and marrow. *Blood* 1996; 88: 472–8.

21. Stewart FM, Zhong S, Wuu J, Hsieh C, Nilsson SK, Quesenberry PJ. Lymphohematopoietic engraftment in minimally myeloablated hosts. *Blood* 1998; 91: 3681–7.

22. Habibian HK, Peters SO, Hsieh CC, Wuu J, Vergilis K, Grimaldi CI, Carlson JE, Frimberger AE, Stewart FM, Quesenberry PJ. The fluctuating phenotype of the lympho-hematopoietic stem cell with cell cycle transit. *J Exp Med* 1998; 188: 393–8.

23. Becker PS, Nilsson SK, Zhifang L, Berrios VM, Dooner MS, Cooper CI, Hsieh CC, Quesenberry PJ. Adhesion receptor expression by hematopoietic cell lines and murine progenitors: Modulation by cytokines and cell cycle status. *Exp Hematol* 1999; 27: 533–41

Tolerance induction using mega-dose stem cell transplants

Y Reisner, MF Martelli

Crossing HLA barriers in leukemia

The use of unseparated peripheral blood transplants after non-myeloablative conditioning in HLA-identical leukemic recipients is associated with a significant alloreactivity. This alloreactivity results from the large number of T-cells in the transplant inoculum which, in most instances, is capable of eradicating the recipient hematopoiesis. This alloreactivity is also associated with a significant incidence of lethal graft-versus-host disease (GVHD). Clearly, while such an outcome may be acceptable for end-stage leukemia patients, the high mortality rates associated with this approach makes its application unfeasible in non-malignant disorders or HLA-mismatched recipients. Therefore, a major challenge is to achieve engraftment of allogeneic hematopoietic cells following non-myeloablative conditioning, in the absence of alloreactive T cells.

The feasibility of 3 loci mismatched transplants from haploidentical family members was first shown in the early 1980s in severe combined immune deficiency (SCID) patients.[1–4] GVHD, which is almost uniformly lethal in such transplants, was completely prevented using 3 log T cell depletion with soybean lectin and E-rosetting. Since then hundreds of patients have been successfully treated with haploidentical T cell-depleted bone marrow from family members.[2–6] Following the encouraging results in SCID patients it was reasonable to assume that in leukemia patients pre-treated with supralethal radiochemotherapy, any remaining immunity would be dramatically reduced, reaching similar levels to those found in SCID patients. It was therefore anticipated that graft rejection should not represent a major problem. However, early results suggested that this was not the case and a high rate of graft rejection was documented.[7–9] Based on murine studies[10–15] which demonstrated the quantitative relationship between the number of host T cells and the number of bone marrow cells required to neutralize the resistance of these cells, we looked for new means to significantly increase the bone marrow cell dose in man. In particular, we hoped to achieve this goal using *ex vivo* expansion. With the advent of granulocyte colony stimulating factor (G-CSF) mobilization in autologous transplants[16,17] it became possible to test the concept of stem cell dose escalation in humans by supplementing bone marrow with peripheral blood progenitor cells (PBPC) collected after administration of G-CSF to the donor. A pilot study carried out between 1993 and 1995 showed for the first time that in humans, as in mice, cell dose escalation facilitated engraftment of T cell-depleted mismatched transplants.[18,19] Subsequently, the extramedullar toxicity of the conditioning protocol was reduced by substituting cyclophosphamide with fludarabine. Moreover, the incidence of GVHD was reduced to < 5% by decreasing the number of T-lymphocytes in the inoculum to a mean of 3 x 10^4/kg, that is, one log less than in the first series of patients. Altogether, our long-term goal to induce high rates of engraftment with low incidences of GVHD and minimal extramedullar toxicity has been achieved.[20,21]

Tolerance induction by human CD34+ hematopoietic progenitor cells

In the first series of leukemia patients receiving 'mega-dose' transplants, the high rate of engraftment could be attributed to several types of accessory cells in the graft, as previously shown in murine models[11,22–30] and *in vitro*.[31,32] The terms 'veto cells' and 'veto activity' were initially used without any allusion to a specific mechanism.[33] Later, several studies began to refer to 'veto cells' as cells capable of destroying cytotoxic T lymphocyte precursors (CTLp) directed specifically against their own class I MHC.[31,34,35] This type of veto activity was shown to be mediated, in the case of CD8-positive veto cells, by the CD8 molecule which can deliver a signal through the alpha 3 domain of a CTLp class I MHC molecule and thus trigger apoptosis of CTLp.

In a second series of leukemia patients, we began to use large doses of purified peripheral blood CD34 cells instead of the entire T cell-depleted transplant, and found there was no reduction in the engraftment rate or the speed of hematopoietic recovery. Cells within the highly CD34-enriched fraction seemed to possess a marked capacity to overcome resistance to engraftment.

To further investigate whether cells within the CD34+ cell fraction are endowed with veto activity, we purified CD34+ cells using the same procedure employed for transplantation in leukemia patients and demonstrated that they are indeed capable of specifically reducing the frequency of CTLp directed against their antigens, but not against stimulator cells of a third party.[36]

After five days of primary mixed leukocyte reaction (MLR) culture in the presence of CD34+ cells, FACS analysis showed that the CD34+ cells were not killed by the alloreactive T-cells. The addition of CD34+ cells to MLR cultures was effective only during the first 48 hours of culture. Thereafter, it seems that the veto effect of these cells was directed at CTLps but did not affect differentiated anti-donor CTLs. IL-2 and IFN-γ production, as measured by intra-cellular staining or by Elispot analysis, are specifically reduced in CD8$^+$ T cells from cultures inhibited by CD34$^+$ cells. Thus, in six experiments we found 70.8% ± 13.1% and 45.2% ± 6.6% inhibition of IL-2 and IFN-γ intracellular levels, respectively. When CD34$^+$ cells were added to MLR against a third party, only a slight inhibition was found ($p < 0.0001$ and $p < 0.017$, respectively). It could be argued that the unique phenotype of cells within the CD34$^+$ compartment lacking B7 might have induced anergy in the responder cells due to inappropriate antigen presentation. However, removal of the CD34$^+$ cells after five days of culture prior to the secondary challenge with the stimulator cells, in the presence of exogenous IL-2, could not reverse the inhibition of anti-donor CTLs. Moreover, addition of anti-CD28 antibody to the primary MLR did not block the inhibition, thus further ruling out an anergy-based mechanism.[37] Recently we found that in mice, early hematopoietic Sca-1$^+$ Lin$^-$ bone marrow cells, similar to human CD34$^+$ cells, are endowed with veto activity.[38] In future, the mechanisms mediating this intriguing activity within the progenitor cell compartment might be identified by taking advantage of different mutant or 'knockout' strains of mice that have impairment of crucial regulatory molecules. Furthermore, if the veto cells within the hematopoietic progenitors are shown to be distinct from the pluripotential hematopoietic stem cells, it might then be more feasible to expand the veto cells *ex vivo*, and use them together with a small number of pluripotential stem cells, for transplantation.

Tolerance induction by mega-dose stem cell transplants in the context of non-myeloablative conditioning

A major question, raised by the finding that CD34 cells are endowed with potent veto activity, is whether it will be possible to use their tolerizing activity in the context of sub-lethal conditioning. Clearly this could be of great importance if it allows induction of tolerance under safe conditions in patients for whom the risk of supralethal radiochemotherapy is not justified, such as in patients with thalassemia, sickle cell anemia and enzyme deficiencies. Furthermore, induction of durable chimerism could be used to induce tolerance as a prelude to organ transplantation.

To answer to this question, we initially used cell dose escalation with T cell-depleted bone marrow.[14] We demonstrated that long-term mixed chimerism, where host and donor type T cells coexist in complete tolerance as judged by limiting dilution analysis for alloreactive CTLs, could be achieved using the mega-dose approach. More recently we showed that donor type chimerism

19

and tolerance can be achieved with dose escalation using purified Sca-1[+]Lin[−] stem cells.[38] As expected, once durable chimerism is achieved, it is possible to induce permanent tolerance for skin grafting. However, this latter study also revealed that a large number of stem cells are required to overcome the host stem cells and T cells remaining after sublethal TBI. Thus, although this study showed in principle the feasibility of using early progenitor cells, it also became apparent that it might be extremely difficult to collect the large numbers required in clinical practice. Therefore, we looked for other sources of veto cells to synergize with the CD34 cells.

Several veto cells have been described[11,22–30] and it seems that the CTLs, as first shown by Miller et al.[31] are among the most potent. However, these cells also possess marked GVH reactivity. Very recently, we developed a new approach to deplete CTLs from alloreactive clones by stimulating the donor T cells against third party stimulators in the absence of exogenous IL-2. This approach is based on the observation that only activated CTLs are capable of surviving IL-2 starvation in primary culture. During the past year we have demonstrated that these non-alloreactive CTLs are endowed with a very potent veto activity.[39,40] To further study the mechanism of action of the veto cells, we used a TCR transgenic mouse model known as 2C. A large proportion of the T cells in 2C mice express the transgene T cell receptor recognising H2[d] and this receptor can be identified using FACS. Thus, the addition of CTLs of H2[d] origin (Balb/c) led to a marked deletion of the transgenic T cells while CTLs from a different source did not.

Most recently we explored the mechanism of action of these potent veto cells.[39,40] Briefly, using FasL deficient mice, gene transfer of FasL into deficient cells and anti-CD8 blocking antibodies we showed that both CD8 and FasL are required for veto activity. Thus, it is possible that CD8 serves to increase the avidity of the T cell receptor so as to bring together the recognizing cell and the veto cell. Once this binding takes place Fas–FasL apoptosis can be triggered. Alternatively, the effect of CD8 could be brought about by some form of signal transduction affecting molecules regulating Fas–FasL apoptosis, such as FLIP.[41]

Finally, when using anti-third party CTLs *in vivo,* we found a marked enhancement of T cell-depleted bone marrow allografts.[39,42] Therefore, it is hoped that engraftment of allogeneic hematopoietic cells following non-myeloablative conditioning, in the absence of alloreactive T cells, might be achieved in patients using 'mega-dose' CD34 stem cells in conjunction with non-alloreactive anti-third party CTLs. We are now testing this approach in a primate model.

References

1. Reisner Y, Kapoor N, Kirkpatrick D, Pollack MS, Cunningham RS, Dupont B, Hodes MZ, Good RA, O'Reilly RJ. Transplantation for severe combined immunodeficiency with HLA-A, B, D, DR incompatible parental marrow cells fractionated by soybean agglutinin and sheep red blood cells. *Blood* 1983; 61: 341–8.

2. Friedrich W, Goldmann SF, Vetter U, Fliedner TM, Heymer B, Peter HH, Reisner Y, Kleihauer E. Immunoreconstitution in severe combined immunodeficiency after transplantation of HLA-haploidentical, T cell-depleted bone marrow. *Lancet* 1984; i: 761–4.

3. Fischer A, Durandy A, de Villartay JP, Vilmer E, Le Deist F, Gerota I, Griscelli C. HLA-Haploidentical bone marrow transplantation for severe combined immune deficiency using E-rosette fractionation and cyclosporine. *Blood* 1986; 67: 444–9.

4. Buckley RH, Schiff SE, Sampson HA, Schiff RI, Markert ML, Knutsen AP, Hershfield MS, Huang AT, Mickey GH, Ward FE. Development of immunity in human severe primary T cell deficiency following haploidentical bone marrow stem cell transplantation. *J Immunol* 1986; 136: 2398–407.

5. Reisner Y, Kapoor N, Kirkpatrick D, Pollack MS, Dupont B, Good RA, O'Reilly RJ. Transplantation for acute leukaemia with HLA-A and B non-identical parental marrow cells fractionated with soybean agglutinin and sheep red blood cells. *Lancet* 1981; ii: 327–31.

6. O'Reilly R, Brochstein J, Collins N, Keever C, Kapoor N, Kirkpatrick D, Kernan N, Dupont B, Burns J, Reisner Y. Evaluation of HLA-haplotype disparate parental marrow grafts depleted of T lymphocytes by differential agglutination with a soybean lectin and E-rosette depletion for the treatment of severe combined immunodeficiency. *Vox Sang* 1986; 51 (Suppl. 2): 81.

7. Gale RP, Reisner Y. Graft rejection and graft-versus-host disease: mirror images. *Lancet* 1986; i: 1468–70.

8. Kernan NA, Flomenberg N, Dupont B, O'Reilly RJ. Graft rejection in recipients of T-cell-depleted HLA-nonidentical marrow transplants for leukemia. Identification of host-derived antidonor allocytotoxic T lymphocytes. *Transplantation* 1987; 43: 842–7.

9. Soiffer RJ, Mauch P, Tarbell NJ, Anderson AS, Freedman AS, Rabinowe SN, Takvorian T, Murray CU, F C, Bosserman L, Dear K, Nadler LM, JR. Total lymphoid irradiation to prevent graft rejection in recipients of HLA non-identical T cell-depleted allogeneic marrow. *Bone Marrow Transplant* 1991; 6: 23–33.

10. Lapidot T, Terenzi A, Singer TS, Salomon O, Reisner Y. Enhancement by dimethyl myleran of donor type chimerism in murine recipients of bone marrow allografts. *Blood* 1989; 73: 2025–32.

11. Lapidot T, Lubin I, Terenzi A, Faktorowich Y, Erlich P, Reisner Y. Enhancement of bone marrow allografts from nude mice into mismatched recipients by T cells void of graft-versus-host activity. *Proc Natl Acad Sci USA* 1990; 87: 4595–9.

12. Uharek L, Gassmann W, Glass B, Steinmann J, Loeffler H, Mueller-Ruchholtz W. Influence of cell dose and graft-versus-host reactivity on rejection rates after allogeneic bone marrow transplantation. *Blood* 1992; 79: 1612–21.

13. Lubin I, Segall H, Marcus H, David M, Kulova L, Steinitz M, Erlich P, Gan J, Reisner Y. Engraftment of human peripheral blood lymphocytes in normal strains of mice. *Blood* 1994; 83: 2368–81.

14. Bachar-Lustig E, Rachamim N, Li HW, Lan F, Reisner Y. Megadose of T cell-depleted bone marrow overcomes MHC barriers in sublethally irradiated mice. *Nat Med* 1995; 1: 1268–73.

15. Bachar-Lustig E, Li HW, Marcus H, Reisner Y. Tolerance induction by megadose stem cell transplants: synergism between SCA-1+ Lin– cells and nonalloreactive T cells. *Transplant Proc* 1998; 30: 4007–8.

16. Sheridan WP, Glenn-Begley C, Juttner CA, Szer J, Bik T, Maher D, McGrath KM, Morstyn G, Fox RM. Effect of peripheral-blood progenitor cells mobilised by filgrastin (G-CSF) on platelet recovery after high-dose chemotherapy. *Lancet* 1992; 339: 640–4.

17. Bensinger W, Singer J, Appelbaum F, Lilleb K, Longin K, Rowley S, Clarke E, Clift R, Hansen J, Shields T, Storb R, Weaver C, Weiden P, Buckner CD. Autologous transplantation with peripheral blood mononuclear cells collected after administration of recombinant granulocyte stimulating factor. *Blood* 1993; 81: 3158–63.

18. Aversa F, Tabilio A, Terenzi A, Velardi A, Falzetti F, Giannoni C, Iacucci R, Zei T, Martelli MP, Gambelunghe C, Rossetti M, Caputo P, Latini P, Aristei C, Raymondi C. Successful engraftment of T-cell-depleted haploidentical "three-loci" incompatible transplants in leukemia patients by addition of recombinant human granulocyte colony-stimulating factor-mobilized peripheral blood progenitor cells to bone marrow inoculum. *Blood* 1994; 84: 3948–55.

19. Reisner Y, Martelli MF. Bone marrow transplantation across HLA barriers by increasing the number of transplanted cells. *Immunol Today* 1995; 16: 437–40.

20. Aversa F, Tabilio A, Velardi A, Cunningham I, Terenzi A, Falzetti F, Ruggeri L, Barbabietola G, Aristei C, Latini P, Reisner Y, Martelli MF. Treatment of high-risk acute leukemia with T-cell-depleted stem cells from related donors with one fully mismatched HLA haplotype. *New Engl J Med* 1998; 339: 1186–93.

21. Reisner Y, Martelli MF. Stem cell escalation enables HLA-disparate haematopoietic transplants in leukaemia patients. *Immunol Today* 1999; 20: 343–7.

22. Lapidot T, Faktorowich Y, Lubin I, Reisner Y. Enhancement of T-cell-depleted bone marrow allografts in the absence of graft-versus-host disease is mediated by CD8+ CD4– and not by CD8– CD4+ thymocytes. *Blood* 1992; 80: 2406–11.

23. Cobbold SP, Martin G, Qin S, Waldmann H. Monoclonal antibodies to promote marrow engraftment and tissue graft tolerance. *Nature* 1986; 323: 164–6.

24. Strober S, Palathumpat V, Schwadron R, Hertel-Wulff B. Cloned natural suppressor cells prevent lethal graft-vs-host disease. *J Immunol* 1987; 138: 699–703.

25. Sugiura K, Inaba M, Ogata H, Yasumizu R, Inaba K, Good RA, Ikehara S. Wheat germ agglutinin-positive cells in a stem cell-enriched fraction of mouse bone marrow have potent natural suppressor activity. *Proc Natl Acad Sci USA* 1988; 85: 4824–6.

26. Tscherning T, Claesson M. Veto-like down regulation of T helper cell reactivity *in vivo* by injection of semi-allogeneic spleen cells. *Immunol Lett* 1991; 29: 223–7.

27. Hiruma K, Nakamura H, Henkart PA, Gress RE. Clonal deletion of postthymic T cells: Veto cells kill precursor cytotoxic T lymphocytes. *J Exp Med* 1992; 175: 863–8.

28. Pierce GE, Watts LM. Do donor cells function as veto cells in the induction and maintenance of tolerance across an MHC disparity in mixed lymphoid radiation chimeras? *Transplantation* 1993; 55: 882–7.

29. Pierce GE, Watts LM. Thy 1+ donor cells function as veto cells in the maintenance of tolerance across a major histocompatibility complex disparity in mixed-lymphoid radiation chimeras. *Transplant Proc* 1993; 25: 331–3.

30. Kaufman CL, Colson YL, Wren SM, Watkins S, Simmons RL, Ildstad ST. Phenotypic characterization of a novel bone marrow-derived cell that facilitates engraftment of allogeneic bone marrow stem cells. *Blood* 1994; 84: 2436–46.

31. Sambhara SR, Miller RG. Programmed cell death of T cells signaled by the T cell receptor and the alpha 3 domain of class I MHC. *Science* 1991; 252: 1424–7.

32. Thomas JM, Carver FM, Cunningham PR, Olson LC, Thomas FT. Kidney allograft tolerance in primates without chronic immunosuppression – the role of veto cells. *Transplantation* 1991; 51: 198–207.

33. Rammensee HG, Nagy ZA, Klein J. Suppression of cell-mediated lymphocytotoxicity against minor histocompatibility antigens mediated by Lyt-1+Lyt-2+ T cells of stimulator-strain origin. *Eur J Immunol* 1982; 12: 930–3.

34. Claesson MH, Miller RG. Functional heterogeneity in allospecific cytotoxic T lymphocyte clones. III. Direct correlation between development of syngeneic cytotoxicity and loss of veto activity; implications for the mechanism of veto action. *Scand J Immunol* 1989; 29: 493–7.

35. Thomas JM, Verbanac KM, Smith JP, Kasten JJ, Gross U, Rebellato LM, Haisch CE, Carver FM, Thomas FT. The facilitating effect of one-DR antigen sharing in renal allograft tolerance induced by donor bone marrow in rhesus monkeys. *Transplantation* 1995; 59: 245–55.

36. Rachamim N, Gan J, Segall H, Krauthgamer R, Marcus H, Berrrebi A, Martelli M, Reisner Y. Tolerance induction by "megadose" hematopoietic transplants: donor-type human CD34 stem cells induce potent specific reduction of host anti-donor cytotoxic T lymphocyte precursors in mixed lymphocyte culture. *Transplantation* 1998; 65: 1386–93.

37. Gur H, Krauthgamer R, Berrebi A, Nagler A, Reisner Y. Specific *in-vitro* inactivation of host anti-donor CTLp by human CD34 progenitor cells: evidence against anergy based mechanisms. *Blood* 1999; 94 (Suppl.): 391a.

38. Bachar-Lustig E, Li HW, Gur H, Krauthgamer R, Marcus H, Reisner Y. Induction of donor-type chimerism and transplantation tolerance across major histocompatibility barriers in sublethally irradiated mice by Sca-1+Lin− bone marrow progenitor cells: synergism with non-alloreactive (Host x Donor)F_1 T cells. *Blood* 1999; 94: 3212–21.

39. Reisner Y, Aversa F, Bachar-Lustig E, Velardi A, Gur H, Tabilio A, Reich-Zeliger S, Krauthgamer R, Martelli MF. The role of megadose CD34 in haploidentical transplantation: potential application to tolerance induction. American Society of Hematology, Education Book, pp. 376, 1999.

40. Reich-Zeliger S, Bachar-Lustig E, Zhao Y, Reisner Y. Enhancement of BM allografts by non-alloreactive donor CTLs: CD8 binding and Fas–FasL apoptosis mediate the veto effect. *Blood* 1999; 94 (Suppl.): 605a.

41. Irmler M, Thome M, Hahne M, Schneider P, Hofmann K, Steiner V, Bodmer JL, Schroter M, Burns K, Mattmann C, Rimoldi D, French LE, Tschopp J. Inhibition of death receptor signals by cellular FLIP. *Nature* 1997; 388: 190–5.

42. Reisner Y, Li HW, Krauthgamer R, Marcus H, Bachar-Lustig E. Non-alloreactive donor anti-third party CTLs facilitaate BM allografts across major histocompatibility barriers in sublethally irradiated mice. *Blood* 1998; 92: 265a.

Mixed chimerism in the treatment of malignant and non-malignant diseases: studies in mice and their clinical application
M Sykes

Mixed chimerism has been developed in animal models as a strategy for inducing tolerance to organ allografts. However, the observation that established mixed chimeras can be converted to full chimeras by administration of donor lymphocyte infusions (DLI), without causing graft-versus-host disease (GVHD),[1] led us to hypothesize that this separation of lymphohematopoietic graft-versus-host (GVH) reactions from clinically significant GVHD could be exploited for the treatment of hematologic malignancies. The subsequent demonstration that non-myeloablative conditioning regimens could be used to achieve mixed chimerism[2,3] led to the development of a modified non-myeloablative regimen designed for the treatment of indolent hematologic malignancies, in which delayed DLI could be used for their immunotherapeutic graft-versus-malignancy (GVM) effect without causing GVHD.[4] Preliminary attempts to apply this approach in patients with aggressive and advanced hematologic malignancies have demonstrated that:

- stable mixed hematopoietic chimerism can be intentionally established, even across HLA barriers, with non-myeloablative host conditioning
- DLI given in an appropriate schedule can convert mixed chimeras to full chimeras and can do so without causing GVHD
- using this approach to induce mixed chimerism can result in powerful GVL effects that may be enhanced by DLI without necessarily causing GVHD.

Advances toward the clinical application of mixed chimerism for the induction of transplantation tolerance

In the mouse model, progress has been made in recent years towards the development of a conditioning regimen for bone marrow transplantation and tolerance induction that is sufficiently non-toxic to be applied clinically. Some of these studies have already been extended to large animal models, and we are hoping to soon see further applications in large animals, followed by extension to the clinical setting. Several years ago Sharabi and Sachs,[2] following on from the work of Cobbold and Waldmann,[5] demonstrated that mixed chimerism and transplantation tolerance could be reliably achieved in mice using a relatively non-toxic, non-myeloablative conditioning regimen. The regimen used low-dose TBI, thymic irradiation and anti-T cell antibodies, followed by fully MHC mismatched allogeneic bone marrow transplantation. Lasting multilineage[2,3] mixed chimerism was achieved, and systemic donor-specific tolerance was evident in both *in vitro*[6] and *in vivo*[2] assays. The major mechanism of tolerance in this model is intrathymic deletion of donor- and host-reactive thymocytes that mature to repopulate the depleted peripheral T cell repertoire.[7–9] Since the depleting anti-CD4 and CD8 monoclonal antibodies given to the recipient are still present in the serum at the time of transplantation, they deplete T cells from donor marrow that could otherwise potentially induce GVHD and deplete host T cells that would otherwise reject the donor marrow. Thus, the animal begins with a 'clean slate' in the peripheral lymphoid tissues. T cells developing in the recipient's thymus after the bone marrow transplant then repopulate the peripheral lymphoid tissues. The central (intrathymic) deletion of donor- and host-reactive thymocytes in these chimeras correlates with the presence of donor- and host-derived class II major histocompatibility complex (MHC)[high] cells in the thymus. The earliest time that both are evident is when T cell regeneration occurs in the thymus.[7] The morphology and distribution of these class II[high] cells suggests that they are dendritic cells and/or macrophages.

In the model discussed above, thymic irradiation is essential to create a 'clean slate' in the thymus, since the anti-T cell monoclonal antibodies used for depletion in the periphery do not effectively eliminate thymocytes,[2] and there are significant numbers of mature alloreactive T cells in the thymic environment of monoclonal antibody/total body irradiation (TBI)-treated mice (B Nikolic and M Sykes, manuscript in preparation). In more recent studies, we have shown that thymic irradiation can be omitted from the protocol using a variety of approaches, including the injection of additional doses of T cell-depleting monoclonal antibodies[3] or, more recently, by giving a single injection of one or another of two costimulatory blockers, anti-CD40L or CTLA4Ig.[10] The potential long-term consequences of thymic irradiation are thereby avoided. Furthermore, we recently showed that both thymic irradiation and recipient T cell depletion can be eliminated by giving a combination of costimulatory blockers along with one injection each of CD40 ligand and CTLA-4Ig. This minimal conditioning regimen has no visible toxicity and avoids the risks that might be associated with prolonged T cell depletion in adults, in whom thymic function is less robust than in children.[11–14] These mice develop lasting mixed chimerism and donor-specific transplantation tolerance by all measures, both *in vivo* and *in vitro*.[15]

Several years ago, we demonstrated that increasing the dose of donor marrow given by approximately 10–13-fold circumvented the need to include low dose

(3 Gy) TBI in our conditioning regimen. Both donor and host T cells were depleted with monoclonal antibodies *in vivo*, simultaneously overcoming both the host-versus-graft (HVG) and the GVH immunologic responses. Thymic irradiation was still required in this regimen to prevent rejection by residual alloreactive thymocytes.[16] Most recently, by combining the high dose marrow approach with costimulatory blockade, we have succeeded in eliminating pre-conditioning altogether. Thus, chimerism can be achieved using a high dose of donor marrow given to mice receiving no TBI, no thymic irradiation and no T cell depletion. Because the host treatment protocol, which involves only costimulatory blockade with anti-CD40L and CTLA4Ig, begins on day 0 when the bone marrow transplant is given, and because tolerance is evident when donor skin is grafted within one day, this protocol is relevant to cadaveric organ transplantation, in which the organ transplant becomes available with little advance notice and must be grafted within a short period of time. With this protocol, lasting mixed chimerism in all lymphoid and myeloid lineages is achieved across full MHC barriers. These mixed chimeras are fully tolerant of the donor; animals with lasting chimerism show donor-specific skin graft acceptance, regardless of whether skin grafting is performed the day after the transplant or weeks or months later.[17] There is no evidence of GVHD in any of these mice, presumably because the smaller number of host-reactive donor T cells in the marrow allograft is exposed to the same immunosuppressive treatment (i.e. costimulatory blockade) as the much larger number of donor-reactive T cells in the host. This protocol advances us considerably towards a completely benign, non-toxic method of bone marrow transplantation for the induction of allograft tolerance.

Application of non-myeloablative induction of mixed chimerism for the treatment of hematologic malignancies

Our belief that the induction of mixed chimerism could be used in the treatment of hematologic malignancies began with work carried out in the mid-1980s. The studies made use of a regimen for induction of permanent mixed chimerism that involved host treatment with lethal TBI and reconstitution with T cell-depleted marrow from the recipient strain and an allogeneic donor strain.[18] In investigating the possible role of recipient-derived suppressor cells to prevent GVHD in such mixed chimeras, we observed that non-tolerant donor lymphocytes could be infused into established mixed chimeras without causing GVHD. The same number of donor T cells would be sufficient to cause rapidly lethal GVHD in a freshly irradiated animal, but the delay of several months prior to DLI appeared to protect these mixed chimeras from GVHD.[1] However, this protection from GVHD did not result from the avoidance of a GVH alloresponse, since the donor T cells in the DLI led to complete elimination of host hematopoiesis, converting the animals from mixed chimeras to full donor-type chimeras.[1] Thus, a powerful GVH response had occurred, but it was not associated with GVHD. The GVH alloresponse appeared to be confined to the lymphohematopoietic system in these animals, and does not affect the epithelial tissues, such as skin, intestine and liver – the usual GVHD target tissues. We have called this GVH alloresponse a 'lymphohematopoietic GVH response' (LGVHR). We are currently investigating the mechanisms that distinguish a LGVHR from one that enters the epithelial GVH target tissues and causes GVHD. We have speculated, based on our experimental observations, that allowing time to pass following lethal conditioning so that the host can recover from tissue injury and inflammation induced by conditioning, makes the T cells given later, which mediate LGVHR, less likely to enter the epithelial tissues and cause GVHD.[1] These observations suggested an attractive approach to treating indolent hematologic malignancies, in which an immediate GVL effect might not be essential, and immunotherapy could be achieved using a DLI given after a sufficient delay, such that the recipient was no longer predisposed to develop GVHD. Since most lymphomas and leukemias reside within the lymphohematopoietic system, the LGHVR induced by DLI might allow the achievement of GVL effects without GVHD. We became particularly aware of the potential of this approach following the development of an effective, reliable non-myeloablative protocol for the induction of mixed chimerism in mice[2] (Figure 1a). A relatively mild, non-toxic conditioning protocol might make BMT available to older patients, who constitute a high proportion of individuals with indolent hematologic malignancies, who cannot readily tolerate a traditional allogeneic transplant regimen. We therefore explored how to achieve a GVL effect using DLI in mice in which mixed chimerism was induced with this non-myeloablative transplantation approach.

We explored BCL1, a spontaneously-derived B cell leukemia from the BALB/c strain, as a model for chronic lymphocytic leukemia (CLL).[19] The results of these studies led us to an important observation: BALB/c mice receiving the non-myeloablative conditioning regimen in Figure 1a, with or without bone marrow transplantation, showed an acceleration of leukemic mortality compared with unconditioned controls. This led us to conclude that the conditioning regimen, which is strongly immunosuppressive but not significantly cytoreductive, suppressed whatever host immunity was available to curtail the growth of the tumor without providing any counterbalancing tumor cytoreduction. We therefore attempted to modify the non-myeloablative conditioning regimen to make it potentially cytoreductive for a variety of hematologic malignancies without increasing its potential toxicity. Toward this

1a. Standard non-myeloablative regimen

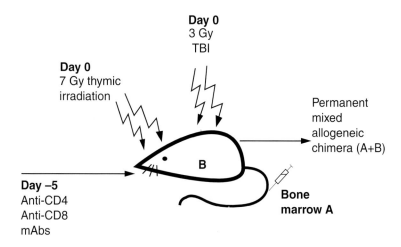

1b. Modified cytoreductive regimen

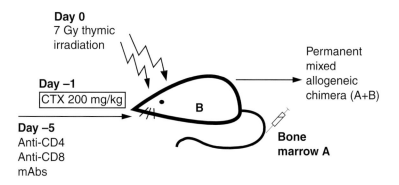

Figure 1. Non-myeloablative regimens for induction of mixed chimerism

goal, we removed TBI from the conditioning and attempted to replace it with various doses of cyclophosphamide (CTX) given on day −1. A dose of 200 mg/kg CTX, given in place of TBI, was found to be sufficient to allow engraftment of fully MHC-mismatched marrow in mice receiving the other components of the non-myeloablative regimen. The modified regimen is shown in Figure 1b. This regimen was non-myeloablative; animals not receiving a transplant after this conditioning treatment survived and demonstrated only transient reductions in leukocyte and platelet counts.[4] The mixed chimerism that was achieved in these animals included a lower proportion of donor cells in all lineages than proportions achieved using the TBI-containing regimen. However, the animals demonstrated chimerism that lasted for the duration of the murine lifespan, and also demonstrated specific tolerance to donor antigens (M Mapara, M Pelot and M Sykes, unpublished data). Similar to the mixed chimerism models discussed above, we found that, when DLI were given to these mixed chimeras 5 weeks post-transplant or even at repeated time points beginning at 5 weeks, the mice became full chimeras. Once again, conversion to full chimerism was not associated with the development of GVHD, as judged by clinical and histological criteria.[4] Thus, in mice receiving bone marrow transplantation with this modified, potentially cytoreductive, non-myeloablative conditioning regimen, LGVHR could occur without causing GVHD.

Principles used in the development of our clinical trial

The observations made in the mouse model described above led us to design a pilot clinical trial for the use of mixed chimerism and DLI to treat patients with refractory hematologic malignancies. A minimally toxic, non-myeloablative conditioning regimen was used to make the protocol applicable to patients who could not tolerate a conventional allogeneic transplant. The regimen included anti-T cell antibodies and thymic irradiation in order to overcome host alloresistance to the donor.

In vivo T cell depletion of donor marrow was accomplished with the same antibody treatment used to deplete recipient T cells. This *in vivo* depletion of the donor marrow inoculum was an important component of our approach, since establishment of a GVHD-free mixed chimeric 'platform' is believed to be essential to allow administration of DLI without inducing GVHD. We hypothesized that the presence of even a low level of GVHD from T cells in the initial marrow inoculum may be sufficient to propagate the pro-inflammatory state in GVHD target tissues that is induced by conditioning therapy, thereby increasing the capacity of DLI to induce GVHD. We believe the absence of GVHD in mice receiving DLI on day 35 reflects the complete absence of even

Day	−5 ► −3	−1	0	+1, +3, +5	35
	CTX 50 mg/kg/day	ATG 20 mg/kg	BMT	ATG 20 mg/kg/day	DLI

7 Gy thymic irradiation   − − − · CSA − − − − − − − − − − ►

Figure 2. Clinical non-myeloablative mixed chimerism protocol

subclinical GVHD prior to that time. The absence of subclinical GVHD results from the complete depletion of donor T cells in the original marrow inoculum by anti-CD4 and CD8 monoclonal antibodies still circulating at the time of transplant. Since similarly effective anti-T cell antibodies are not available for use in humans, we used anti-thymocyte globulin (ATG), which was given both pre- and post-transplant in order to achieve both recipient and donor T cell depletion (Figure 2). Since neither host nor donor T cell depletion is complete using ATG, we also administered a short course of cyclosporine (CSA) beginning on day −1, which was tapered and discontinued before the DLI was given on day 35. Partial tumor cytoreduction may be achieved with CTX. CTX is also used to immunosuppress and myelosuppress the recipient, and thus promote engraftment (Figure 2). DLI was given on day 35 to recipients showing no evidence of GVHD, in the hope of achieving LGVHR for its GVL effect.

While this approach is applicable to the treatment of indolent diseases, in which a delay of 35 days before DLI immunotherapy can be tolerated, we have had to compromise somewhat on this principle in the establishment of a pilot study. Hence, the patients included in this initial study had advanced, chemotherapy-resistant hematologic malignancies of all kinds.

Initial results of the clinical trial

Eligibility criteria included patients with chemorefractory non-Hodgkin's and Hodgkin's lymphoma (NHL and HD), multiple myeloma, acute myelogenous leukemia (AML), acute lymphoblastic leukemia (ALL), CLL and chronic myelogenous leukemia (CML) in blast phase. We accepted up to 2/6 HLA antigen mismatches, and patients aged up to 65 years with reasonable performance status (ECOG 0, 1, 2) and adequate organ function. The early results have recently been published[20,21] so only their highlights are mentioned here.

For the first 21 HLA identical transplants carried out using this protocol, the median age of recipients was 44 years. Eleven patients had NHL, 4 had HD, 4 had acute leukemias and 2 had CLL. Twenty of 21 patients had chemorefractory disease, meaning they could not achieve even a partial remission with chemotherapy, and the remaining patient was in an untreated relapse following autologous transplantation. Three patients had received a prior autologous transplant. Thus, this patient group had malignancies that were at an advanced stage.

DLI was given on day 35 if there was no evidence for or suspicion of GVHD prior to that time. In 11/21 patients there was a suspicion of GVHD by day 35, and these patients did not receive prophylactic DLI. Six of these patients developed acute GVHD (aGVHD), which in all except one patient was grade II and confined to the skin. Among the 7 evaluable patients not receiving prophylactic DLI on day 35, 5 achieved mixed chimerism lasting at least 5 weeks, whereas 2 evaluable patients had lost their graft by 5 weeks. Two patients later received DLI for treatment of relapse and converted to full chimerism. One patient converted spontaneously to full chimerism. It should be noted that loss of the donor marrow graft was not associated with evidence of marrow aplasia, confirming the non-myeloablative nature of the conditioning protocol.

Among the 10 patients who received prophylactic DLI on day 35, some also received a second DLI on day 56, as was originally mandated in our protocol. Of three patients who received two DLIs at 5 and 8 weeks, two developed severe GVHD, so we subsequently removed the 8 week DLI from the protocol. Among recipients of a single DLI, grade $\geq$ II GVHD developed in 3 patients. Grade II GVHD of skin only occurred in two of these patients, and grade III GVHD of the skin and GI tract developed in another. Of 8 evaluable patients receiving one or two prophylactic DLI, 6 converted to full chimerism.

Of the first 20 evaluable patients in this trial, eight achieved complete remission. Of 9 evaluable patients who received prophylactic DLI, 5 achieved a CR, compared with 3/11 who did not receive prophylactic DLI. Although the number of patients in each group is small, a tendency toward more sustained complete remissions in recipients of prophylactic DLI is apparent.

A patient who illustrates the principle that DLI can be associated with conversion to full chimerism without development of GVHD is a 36-year-old man diagnosed in 1992 with stage IV B cell NHL, of follicular mixed small and large cell type. He was initially treated with CHOP, relapsed early, and then underwent autologous peripheral blood stem cell transplantation following high dose TBI and CTX conditioning. He subsequently relapsed, was found to be chemorefractory, and in January 1998 underwent an allogeneic bone marrow transplant from his HLA-matched sibling under the protocol shown in Figure 2. He initially developed mixed chimerism, then received a prophylactic DLI on day 35 and converted to full chimerism without developing GVHD. He has achieved a sustained complete remission of his lymphoma. Thus, DLI can be associated with conversion to full chimerism and potent GVL effects without the development of GVHD, suggesting that in humans, as in mice, GVH reactions can, under certain circumstances, be confined to the lymphohematopoietic system.

The two patients with advanced CLL treated on this protocol have also enjoyed sustained remissions. These remissions were attained gradually following transplant, consistent with an ongoing GVL effect. Thus, the striking anti-tumor responses seen following this novel non-myeloablative preparative regimen in patients with chemorefractory hematologic malignancies, appear to be largely the result of a GVL effect. Most of the patients in this trial had previously received and were resistant to CTX, the only cytoreductive agent used in our conditioning regimen. In patients with easily measurable disease (for example, palpable lymphadenopathy or skin lesions), anti-tumor responses were not maximal until after engraftment had been achieved, or even after DLI.

HLA-mismatched (up to 2/6 HLA-A, B, DR alleles) transplants have been attempted using the protocol in Figure 2. Donor engraftment was achieved in the majority of patients, but usually in association with grade II or III GVHD. Several patients achieved remissions and long-term survival, with long-term mixed or full chimerism and minimal or no ongoing GVHD.[20] However, the initial GVHD necessitated the use of high doses of immunosuppressive therapies in most patients, and precluded the administration of DLI. Therefore, in an effort to better replicate the situation attained in the murine model, in which exhaustive *in vivo* depletion of both donor marrow and host T cells is induced so that GVHD does not develop from the initial marrow transplant, we have recently initiated studies using a more powerful T cell depletion antibody in place of ATG.

In summary

Our data demonstrate that a non-myeloablative transplantation approach is associated with induction of mixed hematopoietic chimerism when either HLA-identical or extensively HLA-mismatched donors are used, and that powerful GVL effects can be achieved against advanced chemotherapy-resistant lymphomas and CLL. Based on these preliminary observations, we predict that this approach might be associated with a high cure rate in patients with indolent hematologic malignancies, especially if they are treated at an early stage, before extremely bulky disease is present. We have hypothesized that the powerful GVL effects observed in our patients may reflect, in part, the ability of non-malignant recipient antigen-presenting cells in mixed chimeras to present recipient alloantigens that more effectively sensitize alloreactive donor T cells than those in full chimeras where the only host hematopoietic cells expressing host alloantigens may be malignant cells. The relatively mild GVHD observed in association with these strong anti-host alloresponses may reflect the relatively lower inflammatory state induced by non-myeloablative compared to standard conditioning. When DLI are given on day 35, the time that has passed since conditioning may have further reduced the tissue inflammation and hence the propensity of GVH-reactive donor T cells to migrate into recipient GVHD target tissues. Studies are currently in progress to address these hypotheses.

Finally, we had the opportunity to study organ allograft tolerance in a patient who had multiple myeloma with associated renal failure, who simultaneously received a kidney and a marrow transplant from her HLA-identical sister in September 1998, using a modification of the protocol in Figure 2. The patient had an uneventful post-transplant course and engrafted on day 12 with 70–90% donor cells. Her mixed chimerism remained stable for 50 days, but decreased continuously after that time, and had disappeared completely by day 105. Remarkably, renal function normalized shortly after transplantation, and no rejection episodes have occurred, despite discontinuation of CSA by day 73. Since then she has not received any immunosuppressive therapy, and renal function remains normal. She has also attained a clinical remission of her multiple myeloma.[22] While it is clear that much remains to be understood about the mechanism of immunological tolerance in this patient and of the remission of her myeloma, the case provides proof of the principle that a relatively benign, well-tolerated non-myeloablative conditioning approach can be used with bone marrow transplantation to induce a state of transplantation tolerance for organ grafts. We plan to carry out more transplants of this nature in the near future in patients who have indications for both a renal and a marrow transplant. Based on these studies and on advances in animal models toward minimizing the toxicity of allogeneic bone marrow transplantation, we are optimistic that non-myeloablative induction of mixed chimerism will become a reliable approach to the induction of transplantation tolerance in the not-too-distant future.

References

1. Sykes M, Sheard MA, Sachs DH. Graft-versus-host-related immunosuppression is induced in mixed chimeras by alloresponses against either host or donor lymphohematopoietic cells. *J Exp Med* 1988; 168: 2391–6.

2. Sharabi Y, Sachs DH. Mixed chimerism and permanent specific transplantation tolerance induced by a non-lethal preparative regimen. *J Exp Med* 1989; 169: 493–502.

3. Tomita Y, Sachs DH, Khan A, Sykes M. Additional mAb injections can replace thymic irradiation to allow induction of mixed chimerism and tolerance in mice receiving bone marrow transplantation after conditioning with anti-T cell mAbs and 3 Gy whole body irradiation. *Transplantation* 1996; 61: 469–77.

4. Pelot MR, Pearson DA, Swenson K, Zhao G, Sachs J, Yang Y-G, Sykes M. Lymphohematopoietic graft-versus-host reactions can be induced without graft-versus-host disease in murine mixed chimeras established with a cyclophosphamide-based non-myeloablative conditioning regimen. *Biol Blood Marrow Transplant* 1999; 5: 133–43.

5. Cobbold SP, Martin G, Qin S, Waldmann H. Monoclonal antibodies to promote marrow engraftment and tissue graft tolerance. *Nature* 1986; 323: 164–5.

6. Sharabi Y, Abraham VS, Sykes M, Sachs DH. Mixed allogeneic chimeras prepared by a non-myeloablative regimen: requirement for chimerism to maintain tolerance. *Bone Marrow Transplant* 1992; 9: 191–7.

7. Tomita Y, Khan A, Sykes M. Role of intrathymic clonal deletion and peripheral anergy in transplantation tolerance induced by bone marrow transplantation in mice conditioned with a non-myeloablative regimen. *J Immunol* 1994; 153: 1087–98.

8. Khan A, Tomita Y, Sykes M. Thymic dependence of loss of tolerance in mixed allogeneic bone marrow chimeras after depletion of donor antigen. Peripheral mechanisms do not contribute to maintenance of tolerance. *Transplantation* 1996; 62: 380–7.

9. Manilay JO, Pearson DA, Sergio JJ, Swenson KG, Sykes M. Intrathymic deletion of alloreactive T cells in mixed bone marrow chimeras prepared with a nonmyeloablative conditioning regimen. *Transplantation* 1998; 66: 96–102.

10. Wekerle T, Sayegh MH, Ito H, Hill J, Chandraker A, Pearson DA, Swenson KG, Zhao G, Sykes M. Anti-CD154 or CTLA4Ig obviates the need for thymic irradiation in a non-myeloablative conditioning regimen for the induction of mixed hematopoietic chimerism and tolerance. *Transplantation* 1999; 68: 1348–55.

11. Berzins SP, Boyd RL, Miller JFAP. The role of the thymus and recent thymic migrants in the maintenance of the adult peripheral lymphocyte pool. *J Exp Med* 1998; 187: 1839–48.

12. Hakim FT, Cepeda R, Kaimei S, Mackall CL, McAtee N, Zukewski J, Cowan K, Gress RE. Constraints on CD4 recovery postchemotherapy in adults: Thymic insufficiency and apoptotic decline of expanded peripheral CD4 cells. *Blood* 1997; 90: 3789–98.

13. Jamieson BD, Douek DC, Killian S, Hultin LE, Scripture-Adamas DD, Giorgi JV, Marelli D, Koup RA, Zack JA. Generation of functional thymocytes in the human adult. *Immunity* 1999; 10: 569–75.

14. Poulin J-F, Viswanathan MN, Harris JM, Komanduri KV, Wieder E, Ringuette N, Jenkins M, McCune JM, Sekaly R-P. Direct evidence for thymic function in adult humans. *J Exp Med* 1999; 190: 479–86.

15. Wekerle T, Sayegh MH, Hill J, Zhao Y, Chandraker A, Swenson KG, Zhao G, Sykes M. Extrathymic T cell deletion and allogeneic stem cell engraftment induced with costimulatory blockade is followed by central T cell tolerance. *J Exp Med* 1998; 187: 2037–44.

16. Sykes M, Szot GL, Swenson K, Pearson DA. Induction of high levels of allogeneic hematopoietic reconstitution and donor-specific tolerance without myelosuppressive conditioning. *Nat Med* 1997; 3: 783–7.

17. Wekerle T, Kurtz J, Ito H, Ronquillo JV, Dong V, Zhao G, Shaffer J, Sayegh MH, Sykes M. Allogeneic bone marrow transplantation with costimulatory blockade induces macrochimerism and tolerance without cytoreductive host treatment. *Nat Med* 2000; 6: 464–9.

18. Ildstad ST, Sachs DH. Reconstitution with syngeneic plus allogeneic or xenogeneic bone marrow leads to specific acceptance of allografts or xenografts. *Nature* 1984; 307: 168–70.

19. Slavin S, Strober S. Spontaneous murine B-cell leukemia. *Nature* 1978; 272: 624–6.

20. Sykes M, Preffer F, McAfee S, Saidman SL, Colby C, Sackstein R, Sachs DH, Spitzer TR. Mixed lymphohematopoietic chimerism and graft-vs-lymphoma effects are achievable in adult humans following non-myeloablative therapy and HLA-mismatched donor bone marrow transplantation. *Lancet* 1999; 353: 1755–9.

21. Spitzer TR, McAfee S, Sackstein R, Colby C, Toh HC, Multani P, Saidman S, Weymouth D, Preffer F, Poliquin C, Foley A, Cox B, Dombkowski D, Andrews D, Sachs DH, Sykes M. The intentional induction of mixed chimerism and achievement of anti-tumor responses following non-myeloablative conditioning therapy and HLA-matched and mismatched donor bone marrow transplantation for refractory hematologic malignancies. *Biol Blood Marrow Transplant* 2000; 6: 309–20.

22. Spitzer TR, Delmonico F, Tolkoff-Rubin N, McAfee S, Sackstein R, Saidman S, Colby C, Sykes M, Sachs DH, Cosimi AB. Combined HLA-matched donor bone marrow and renal transplantation for multiple myeloma with end stage renal disease: The induction of allograft tolerance through mixed lymphohematopoietic chimerism. *Transplantation* 1999; 68: 480–4.

Post-transplant immunosuppression – canine models and clinical application

BM Sandmaier, PA McSweeney, D Niederwieser, DG Maloney, KG Blume, A Molina, J Shizuru, T Chauncey, G Georges, JM Zaucha, M Maris, A Woolfrey, R Storb

Introduction

Allogeneic hematopoietic stem cell transplantation (HSCT) has emerged as a treatment option for both malignant and non-malignant hematologic diseases. The intensive cytotoxic conditioning regimens used in conjunction with conventional HSCT are aimed both at eradicating the underlying disease and suppressing the host immune system to prevent rejection of the allograft. The stem cell graft both rescues the recipient from otherwise lethal marrow toxicity caused by the conditioning regimens and eliminates residual host resistance and tumor cells via graft-versus-host (GVH) reactions. Post-grafting immunosuppression controls graft-versus-host disease (GVHD) and attempts to establish long-term graft tolerance. Widespread application of stem cell transplantation has been limited by complications related to the conditioning regimens. The regimens' intensities have been escalated to the point where organ toxicities are common, resulting in morbidity and mortality and, thus, restricting the use of transplantation to relatively young patients at most transplant centers. As it is known that both host-versus-graft (HVG) and GVH reactions are mediated by T cells in the major histocompatibility complex (MHC)-identical setting, we reasoned that agents aimed at controlling GVHD after transplant could be substituted for some or even all of the myeloablative therapy customarily given before transplant. Accordingly, preclinical studies have been carried out to develop optimal post-grafting immunosuppression capable of controlling both HVG and GVH reactions. The present report reviews the preclinical studies and describes their clinical translation.

Canine models of non-myeloablative HSCT

Many of the clinical HSCT protocols used in Seattle were developed in a random bred dog model over the past 35 years.[1–3] Total body irradiation (TBI) was an integral part of many of the early conventional conditioning regimens and has also played an important role in the development of newer non-myeloablative transplantation (NST) approaches. In the absence of marrow rescue, a TBI dose of 400 cGy delivered at 7 cGy/min is lethal in dogs, with 27 of 28 dogs dying from problems related to prolonged pancytopenia.[4] At 200 cGy TBI, only 1 of 19 dogs died, with the remainder showing spontaneous hematopoietic recovery. At the myeloablative TBI dose of 450 cGy, two commonly used immunosuppressive GVHD prevention drugs, cyclosporine (CSA) and prednisone, were tested separately for their ability to facilitate engraftment. CSA was given at a dose of 15 mg/kg b.i.d. p.o., days –1 to 35. All of the CSA-treated animals had stable donor engraftment compared to only a minority of dogs not given CSA ($p = 0.01$).[5] If the CSA was given before transplant, there was no effect on promoting stable donor engraftment. Prednisone was administered at 12.5 mg/kg orally b.i.d. on days –5 to 3, with subsequent tapering of the dose through day 32. The high-dose prednisone was completely ineffective with none of the dogs having sustained engraftment. When the TBI dose was lowered to the sublethal range of 200 cGy, the use of post-transplant CSA alone failed to achieve stable engraftment. To evaluate whether engraftment could be improved with the use of combination therapy, the antimetabolite methotrexate (MTX) was added to CSA, since previous data showed synergism of these two agents for GVHD prophylaxis in both dogs and human patients. Of five dogs studied, two engrafted as mixed chimeras and three rejected their grafts. A novel immunosuppressive drug, mycophenolate mofetil (MMF), was also tested in this model. Previous data had indicated that MMF/CSA was superior to MTX/CSA for GVHD prophylaxis.[6] Consistent with those data, only one of 11 dogs studied rejected its allograft after 12 weeks, whereas 10 dogs became mixed chimeras for up to 130 weeks after transplant without evidence of GVHD.[7] Mixed chimerism was stable in all dogs for as long as they were followed. When the dose of TBI was lowered to 100 cGy, all six MMF/CSA-treated dogs rejected their marrow grafts within 3–12 weeks of transplantation, indicating that 100 cGy was below the threshold of pretransplant immunosuppression needed to achieve sustained engraftment. A recent study involving additional treatment with the T-cell co-stimulation blocker CTLA4-Ig, in the presence of donor antigen, demonstrated that sustained engraftment was possible after 100 cGy TBI.[8] Other evidence supporting the role of immunosuppression in the induction of mixed chimerism has been obtained through studies of a monoclonal antibody (mAb) directed at the TCRαβ complex. Antibody given from day –1 to day 7 facilitated stable donor engraftment in five of six dogs after 450 cGy TBI,[9] therefore controlling HVG reactions in a manner that was comparable to that seen with CSA given for 35 days after transplant.[5] Data to support the hypothesis that the major role of the pretransplant TBI was to provide host immunosuppression and not to create 'marrow space' were provided in an experiment where MMF/CSA-treated dogs given 450 cGy radiation limited to cervical, thoracic, and upper abdominal lymph nodes had successful engraftment of DLA-identical littermate marrow.[10]

We were unable to convert mixed stable hematopoietic chimerism to full donor chimerism in dogs using unmodified donor lymphocyte infusions (DLI). This becomes relevant when considering that mixed hematopoietic chimerism may not be sufficient to induce a cure of an underlying hematopoietic malignancy. Therefore, a protocol was developed whereby canine marrow donors were sensitized with skin grafts from recipients, then peripheral blood mononuclear cells were harvested from the donors and given to the recipients. Three to five weeks after infusion all recipients converted to > 95% donor chimerism.[11] Current studies are attempting to identify ways of achieving *in vitro* sensitization that can be translated to human patients.

In the MHC non-identical setting, the barriers to engraftment are more complex and difficult to overcome. Whereas in the MHC identical setting T cells mediate both HVG and GVH reactions, in the MHC non-identical setting natural killer (NK) cells are important effectors of graft rejection in addition to T cells. In dogs given marrow infusions from DLA-mismatched unrelated donors, engraftment was uniformly seen after conditioning with 1800 cGy TBI, was the exception after a single dose of 920 cGy, and was never seen with lower TBI doses.[12] When cytokine (granulocyte colony stimulating factor [G-CSF] or G-CSF/SCF) mobilized peripheral blood stem cells (PBSC) were substituted for marrow, all MHC haploidentical littermates had successful allogeneic engraftment after 920 cGy TBI.[13] The findings made with cytokine mobilized PBSC resemble those made previously in MHC-mismatched recipients given marrow supplemented by peripheral blood buffy coat cells, which resulted in 95% engraftment.[12] Alternatively, an anti-CD44 mAb, S5, was shown to promote engraftment of marrow in MHC-mismatched unrelated dogs not given additional buffy coat infusions after 920 cGy TBI.[14–16] CD44 is a cellular adhesion molecule expressed on virtually all hematopoietic cells and also on other non-hematopoietic cells. CD44 function is related to both homotypic and heterotypic cell–cell interactions, along with adhesion to the cellular matrix. CD44 also plays a role in cell activation. The anti-CD44 mAb S5 has been shown to increase NK activity,[17] and this is accomplished through an increase in effector–target conjugate formation and elaboration of TNFα that is independent of monocytes.[18] Also, binding of S5 increases radiation sensitivity of NK cells both *in vitro* and *in vivo*. Currently, we are studying the feasibility of NST in DLA haploidentical littermates. When the anti-CD44 mAb, S5, was given before conditioning with 450 cGy TBI, and MMF/CSA was administered after transplant, all dogs showed initial allogeneic engraftment, and only a small number of dogs subsequently rejected their graft.[19] The result was significantly better than that seen in controls not given mAb S5 combined with postgrafting MMF and CSA. When the TBI dose was lowered to 200 cGy all animals initially engrafted, although half later rejected.[19] Current studies are evaluating whether extending the duration of postgrafting immunosuppression decreases the incidence of late graft rejection.

Severe canine hereditary hemolytic anemia due to pyruvate kinase deficiency can be corrected using HSCT transplants from healthy littermates following conventional high-dose conditioning regimens.[20,21] The disease is an ideal model in which to test the hypothesis that mixed chimerism can correct the phenotypic manifestations of certain genetic diseases. A five-year-old Basenji dog with pyruvate kinase deficiency was given 200 cGy TBI before, and MMF/CSA after, a marrow transplant from a healthy MHC-identical littermate.[22] Before transplant, the dog was severely anemic and had a high reticulocyte count. When the animal engrafted with donor cells, both the reticulocyte counts and hematocrit normalized and hematopoiesis was 85% donor. However the LDH remained elevated indicating ongoing hemolysis. Consequently, the pre-existing hemosiderosis and liver cirrhosis worsened, and the dog died more than a year after transplant from liver failure. This information is important when designing treatment for patients with non-malignant diseases using NST. Individuals transplanted for hemolytic diseases may need conversion to complete chimerism while others, e.g. those with sickle cell disease, may benefit from mixed chimerism.

Further studies in both the DLA-identical and haploidentical dogs are ongoing, evaluating more effective non-toxic pregrafting immunosuppression. Other important questions concern the duration of postgrafting immunosuppression as this may be relevant for preventing late graft rejections, and additionally, for better control of GVHD. The timing, dosing, effectiveness and safety of DLI are also being investigated as is the use of short-lived alpha-emitting radionuclide (Bi-213) conjugates with anti-CD45 and anti-CD3/TCR$\alpha\beta$ mAbs to provide targeted immunosuppression.

The results of the preclinical canine studies formed the basis of a new conceptual scheme for allogeneic HSCT in humans, and early clinical results indicate the approach is both feasible and successful.

Clinical results

The new conceptual scheme involved outpatient allogeneic HSCT for patients with hematologic malignancies who were older than 50 years, or who were ineligible for conventional HSCT because of medical comorbidities.[23–25] Patients were given 200 cGy TBI, delivered as a single fraction at 8 cGy/min, and postgrafting immunosuppression consisting of CSA 6.25 mg/kg b.i.d. orally from day –1 to day 35, then tapered off by day 56 (initial patients had CSA discontinued on day 35 without a taper), and MMF given at 15 mg/kg b.i.d. orally from days 0–27. The patients received G-CSF mobilized PBSC from HLA-identical sibling donors on day 0. Chimerism analyses were carried out on days 28, 56, and 84. Over 50 patients have been treated on this protocol at the Fred Hutchinson Cancer Research Center, Seattle Veterans Administration Hospital, Stanford University, and the University of Leipzig. The median age of patients was 56 years. Over half of the patients were treated entirely in the outpatient setting for the first 2 months post-transplant, and the remainder had a median hospital stay of 8 days. None of the patients experienced regimen-related alopecia, mucositis, diarrhea, or venocclusive disease of the liver. The median number of platelet transfusions required during the first 60 days was zero and the median number of red blood cell transfusions was two. All patients showed mixed donor–host or full-donor hematopoietic chimerism by day 28. The highest degree of donor engraftment was seen in patients with preceding autologous transplants and/or a history of intensive chemotherapy.[26] Overall, 20% of patients rejected their allografts. The degree of donor T cell chimerism was predictive of graft rejection, with patients who showed < 50% donor T-cell chimerism on day 28 experiencing the highest risk of rejection.[26] All patients who rejected their graft returned to baseline hematologic status. Approximately 40% of patients developed grade II–IV acute GVHD that was readily controlled with either resumption of CSA or the addition of corticosteroids.[27] The regimen-related mortality was 6.8%, though follow-up was short. Among the first 44 patients, major disease responses were observed in 70% of those with measurable disease before transplant. This included all four patients with chronic myelogenous leukemia (CML), five of seven with chronic lymphocytic leukemia (CLL), one with acute myeloid leukemia, one with acute lymphoblastic leukemia, two of five with multiple myeloma, two of four with Hodgkin's disease, and one of three with non-Hodgkin's lymphoma. Four patients with CML and two with CLL achieved complete molecular remissions (as assessed using polymerase chain reaction [PCR] analysis). While follow-up was too short to assess durability of the anti-tumor responses, the preliminary data indicated that acute toxicities in this elderly patient population was minimal, allowing the transplants to be done mainly in the ambulatory care setting. Modifications to the immunosuppression in order to enhance engraftment and reduce GVHD will mean this procedure could be carried out safely in a large number of patients. The results in HLA-identical siblings have prompted us to investigate the use of these transplants in other clinical settings including HSCT from HLA-matched unrelated donors.

References

1.   Deeg HJ, Storb R. Canine marrow transplantation models. *Curr Topics Vet Res* 1994; 1: 103–14.

2.   Georges GE, Sandmaier BM, Storb R. Animal models. In: Reiffers J, Goldman J, Armitage J (eds): *Blood Stem Cell Transplantation*. London: Martin Dunitz Publishers, pp. 1–17, 1998.

3.   Wagner JL, Storb R. Preclinical large animal models for hematopoietic stem cell transplantation. *Curr Opin Hematol* 1996; 3: 410–5.

4.   Storb R, Raff RF, Graham T, Appelbaum FR, Deeg HJ, Schuening FG, Shulman H, Pepe M. Marrow toxicity of fractionated versus single dose total body irradiation is identical in a canine model. *Int J Radiat Oncol Biol Phys* 1993; 26: 275–83.

5.   Yu C, Storb R, Mathey B, Deeg HJ, Schuening FG, Graham TC, Seidel K, Burnett R, Wagner JL, Shulman H, Sandmaier BM. DLA-identical bone marrow grafts after low-dose total body irradiation: Effects of high-dose corticosteroids and cyclosporine on engraftment. *Blood* 1995; 86: 4376–81.

6.   Yu C, Seidel K, Nash RA, Deeg HJ, Sandmaier BM, Barsoukov A, Santos E, Storb R. Synergism between mycophenolate mofetil and cyclosporine in preventing graft-versus-host disease among lethally irradiated dogs given DLA-nonidentical unrelated marrow grafts. *Blood* 1998; 91: 2581–7.

7.   Storb R, Yu C, Wagner JL, Deeg HJ, Nash RA, Kiem H-P, Leisenring W, Shulman H. Stable mixed hematopoietic chimerism in DLA-identical littermate dogs given sublethal total body irradiation before and pharmacological immunosuppression after marrow transplantation. *Blood* 1997; 89: 3048–54.

8.   Storb R, Yu C, Zaucha JM, Deeg HJ, Georges G, Kiem H-P, Nash RA, McSweeney PA, Wagner JL. Stable mixed hematopoietic chimerism in dogs given donor antigen, CTLA4Ig, and 100 cGy total body irradiation before and pharmacologic immunosuppression after marrow transplant. *Blood* 1999; 94: 2523–9.

9.   Barsoukov AA, Moore PF, Storb R, Santos EB, Sandmaier BM. The use of an anti-TCRαβ monoclonal antibody to control host-versus-graft reactions in canine marrow allograft recipients conditioned with low dose total body irradiation. *Transplantation* 1999; 67: 1329–35.

10. Storb R, Yu C, Barnett T, Wagner JL, Deeg HJ, Nash RA, Kiem H-P, McSweeney P, Seidel K, Georges G, Zaucha JM. Stable mixed hematopoietic chimerism in dog leukocyte antigen-identical littermate dogs given lymph node irradiation before and pharmacologic immunosuppression after marrow transplantation. *Blood* 1999; 94: 1131–6.

11. Georges GE, Storb R, Thompson JD, Yu C, Gooley T, Bruno B, Nash RA. Adoptive immunotherapy in canine mixed chimeras after nonmyeloablative hematopoietic cell transplantation. *Blood* 2000; 95: 3262–9.

12. Storb R, Deeg HJ. Failure of allogeneic canine marrow grafts after total body irradiation: Allogeneic 'resistance' vs transfusion induced sensitization. *Transplantation* 1986; 42: 571–80.

13. Sandmaier BM, Storb R, Santos EB, Krizanac-Bengez L, Lian T, McSweeney PA, Yu C, Schuening FG, Deeg HJ, Graham T. Allogeneic transplants of canine peripheral blood stem cells mobilized by recombinant canine hematopoietic growth factors. *Blood* 1996; 87: 3508–13.

14. Sandmaier BM, Storb R, Appelbaum FR, Gallatin WM. An antibody that facilitates hematopoietic engraftment recognizes CD44. *Blood* 1990; 76: 630–5.

15. Schuening F, Storb R, Goehle S, Meyer J, Graham TC, Deeg HJ, Appelbaum FR, Sale GE, Graf L, Loughran TP, Jr. Facilitation of engraftment of DLA-nonidentical marrow by treatment of recipients with monoclonal antibody directed against marrow cells surviving radiation. *Transplantation* 1987; 44: 607–13.

16. Sandmaier BM, Storb R, Bennett KL, Appelbaum FR, Santos EB. Epitope specificity of CD44 for monoclonal antibody dependent facilitation of marrow engraftment in a canine model. *Blood* 1998; 91: 3494–502.

17. Tan PHS, Santos EB, Rossbach HC, Sandmaier BM. Enhancement of natural killer activity by an antibody to CD44. *J Immunol* 1993; 150: 812–20.

18. Tan PH, Liu Y, Santos EB, Sandmaier BM. Mechanisms of enhancement of natural killer activity by an antibody to CD44: Increase in conjugate formation and release of tumor necrosis factor α. *Cell Immunol* 1995; 164: 255–64.

19. Sandmaier BM, Yu C, Gooley T, Santos EB, Storb R. Haploidentical stem cell allografts after nonmyeloablative therapy in a preclinical large animal model. *Blood* 1999; 94 (Suppl. 1): 318a.

20. Weiden PL, Storb R, Graham TC, Schroeder ML. Severe hereditary haemolytic anaemia in dogs treated by marrow transplantation. *Br J Haematol* 1976; 33: 357–62.

21. Weiden PL, Hackman RC, Deeg HJ, Graham TC, Thomas ED, Storb R. Long-term survival and reversal of iron overload after marrow transplantation in dogs with congenital hemolytic anemia. *Blood* 1981; 57: 66–70.

22. Yu C, Nash R, Lothrop C, Zaucha J, Storb R. Severe canine hereditary hemolytic anemia treated by marrow grafts using nonmyeloablative immunosuppression. *Blood* 1998; 92 (Suppl. 1): 263a.

23. McSweeney PA, Wagner JL, Maloney DG, Radich J, Shizuru J, Bensinger WI, Bryant E, Chauncey TR, Flowers MED, Kauffman M, Minor CS, Nash RA, Blume K, Storb R. Outpatient PBSC allografts using immunosuppression with low-dose TBI before, and cyclosporine (CSP) and mycophenolate mofetil (MMF) after transplant. *Blood* 1998; 92 (Suppl. 1): 519a.

24. Storb R. Nonmyeloablative preparative regimens: experimental data and clinical practice. In: Perry MC (ed.), *ASCO Education Book*. pp. 241–9, 1999.

25. Storb R, Yu C, McSweeney P. Mixed chimerism after transplantation of allogeneic hematopoietic cells. In: Thomas ED, Blume KG, Forman SJ (eds), *Hematopoietic Cell Transplantation*, 2nd Edition. Boston: Blackwell Science, 1999, pp. 287–95.

26. Molina A, McSweeney P, Maloney DG, Sandmaier B, Wagner JL, Nash R, Chauncey T, Bryant E, Storb R. Degree of early donor T-cell chimerism predicts GVHD and graft rejection in patients with nonmyeloablative hematopoietic stem cell allografts. *Blood* 1999; 94 (Suppl. 1): 394a.

27. McSweeney P, Niederwieser D, Shizuru J, Molina A, Wagner J, Minor S, Radich J, Chauncey T, Hegenbart U, Maloney D, Nash R, Sandmaier B, Blume K, Storb R. Outpatient allografting with minimally myelosuppressive, immunosuppressive conditioning of low-dose TBI and postgrafting cyclosporine (CSP) and mycophenolate mofetil (MMF). *Blood* 1999; 94 (Suppl. 1): 393a.

New frontiers in cancer therapy

Non-myeloablative stem cell transplantation (NST)

Section 2 – Clinical studies

Non-myeloablative preparative regimens and allogeneic hematopoietic cellular transplantation for induction of graft-versus-malignancy effects

R Champlin

Allogeneic bone marrow transplantation was initially considered as a means to deliver supralethal doses of chemotherapy and total body irradiation for the treatment of malignancy.[1,2] The marrow transplant was considered a supportive care modality to restore hematopoiesis. Considerable data indicate, however, that high-dose therapy does not eradicate the malignancy in most patients, and that much of the therapeutic benefit of allogeneic marrow transplantation is related to a graft-versus-malignancy (GVM) effect mediated by donor derived immunocompetent cells. An alternative strategy is emerging using allogeneic transplant not as a means to deliver high-dose therapy, but as a method to induce GVM effects as primary therapy.

Donor lymphocyte infusions

The data supporting the existence of a GVM effect is summarized in Table 1. The most direct evidence is the ability of donor lymphocyte infusions (DLI) to reinduce remission in patients with recurrent malignancy after allogeneic hematopoietic transplantation. The malignancy typically recurs in host-derived cells, but residual normal hematopoiesis and immunity are donor derived. The infused donor lymphocytes are, therefore, not rejected, but graft-versus-host disease (GVHD) and GVM effects may develop. The most extensive studies of DLI have been carried out in patients with recurrent chronic myelogenous leukemia (CML). Approximately 70% of patients recurring into chronic phase

Table 1. Clinical evidence supporting an allogeneic GVM effect against hematologic malignancies

- Demonstration of reactivity of donor derived T-cell clones against malignant cells
- Minimal residual disease after allografts is slowly eliminated in T-cell replete transplants
- Reduced risk of relapse in patients with GVHD
- Increased risk of relapse after syngeneic or T-cell depleted transplants
- Induction of remission by DLI in patients relapsing post-transplant
- Induction of remission after non-ablative preparative regimen

achieve complete remission after DLI. There is initially little change in peripheral blood counts following DLI, but leukemic cells are eliminated after a median of four months followed by recovery of donor-derived hematopoiesis.[3–5] Antileukemic effectors presumably proliferate *in vivo* following the infusion and must reach a threshold level to eradicate the leukemia. Normal host derived hematopoietic cells are also eliminated.[6] Marrow aplasia may occur unless sufficient donor derived normal progenitors are present to restore hematopoiesis.[7,8]

Non-myeloablative preparative regimens

The high dose chemotherapy and radiation typically used as the preparative regimen for blood stem cell or bone marrow transplantation produces considerable morbidity and mortality. This approach must therefore be restricted to young patients without comorbidities. The majority of patients with hematologic malignancies are not eligible for high-dose therapy because of older age or comorbid conditions. An alternate strategy is to use a less intensive preparative regimen designed not to eradicate the malignancy but to provide sufficient immunosuppression to achieve engraftment of an allogeneic blood stem cell or marrow graft, thus allowing the development of an immune GVM effect.

These reduced toxicity regimens are frequently termed non-myeloablative. As a working definition, a truly non-myeloablative regimen should allow relatively prompt hematopoietic recovery (< 28 days) without a transplant, and mixed chimerism usually occurs upon engraftment following hematopoietic transplantation. These lower dose preparative regimens do not ablate host immunity and depend on the activity of donor T-cells to achieve engraftment. Initial studies focused on patients with an HLA-identical sibling. More intensive regimens are required for engraftment in settings of greater genetic disparity including unrelated donor transplants and in HLA-non-identical donor–recipient pairs.[1]

We and others have evaluated this non-myeloablative transplant strategy (NST).[9–13] The treatment scheme is illustrated in Figure 1. The 'non-ablative' regimen does not completely eliminate host-derived cells, but allogeneic T-cells react against and then eradicate residual host derived normal hematopoietic cells and the malignancy. This process takes months to complete and patients may receive additional donor lymphocytes as necessary to augment the GVM effects. This approach reduces drug toxicity and may also reduce the risk of severe acute GVHD, since the clinical manifestations of GVHD partly result from the toxicity of the preparative regimen and subsequent cytokine release in addition to the alloreactivity of the graft.[14,15] Infectious complications could

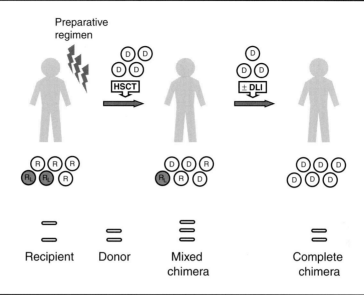

Figure 1. Scheme for non-ablative hematopoietic transplantation. Recipients (R) receive a relatively non-toxic preparative regimen designed primarily to achieve engraftment of an allogeneic hematopoietic cell transplant for the purpose of inducing a GVM effect. A short course immunosuppressive treatment is given to prevent GVHD. Initially mixed chimerism is present, thus there is coexistence of donor (D) cells with recipient-derived normal (R) and leukemia (R$_L$) cells. Recipient and donor patterns of restriction fragment length polymorphisms are shown. Donor-derived T cells act to eradicate residual recipient-derived normal and malignant hematopoietic cells leading to complete chimerism and remission. DLI may be administered to enhance GVM effects

also be reduced, since the non-ablative preparative regimen does not completely eliminate host derived immunocompetent cells.

Disease susceptibility to GVM

There are major differences between diseases in susceptibility to GVM effects, and hence sensitivity to NST (see Table 2). CML and indolent B-cell malignancies appear to be most sensitive. In CML, T-cell depleted transplants are associated with a 5-fold increase in the risk of relapse.[16–20] Minimal residual disease can be detected early post-transplant in the majority of patients with CML using cytogenetic or polymerase chain reaction-based techniques.[21–30] Malignant cells are usually undetectable 6 months post-transplant in patients receiving unmodified (T-cell replete) marrow transplants, presumably because of a GVM effect. Approximately 70% of CML patients relapsing into chronic phase achieve complete remission if they receive a DLI from the original transplant donor.[3,5,31–35] The best results are seen if the DLI is given early in the course of relapse.[8,36] In responders, residual leukemia becomes undetectable

Table 2. Disease sensitivity to GVM effects

Sensitive	Intermediate	Insensitive
CML	AML	ALL
Low-grade lymphoma	Intermediate-grade lymphoma	High-grade lymphoma
Mantle cell lymphoma	Multiple myeloma	
CLL	Hodgkin's disease	

by polymerase chain reaction analysis for bcr-abl rearrangement and these responses are generally durable.

Relatively few patients have received allogeneic transplants for indolent lymphoid malignancies (low-grade lymphoma and chronic lymphocytic leukemia [CLL]), but available data indicate that potent GVM effects occur against these disorders. Selected patients with CLL[37] or lymphoma[38–42] have also responded to DLI or modifications of immunosuppressive therapy. These data have led to trials of non-ablative allogeneic transplants using a low-dose immunosuppressive preparative regimen to achieve engraftment; in preliminary studies many patients with low-grade lymphoma, mantle cell lymphoma or CLL have achieved durable remissions.[43,44]

A second group of malignancies including acute myelogenous leukemia (AML), multiple myeloma, Hodgkin's disease (HD) and intermediate-grade lymphoma have intermediate sensitivity to GVM effects. Patients with AML have a 3-fold increased risk of relapse following syngeneic transplants compared to transplants from HLA-identical siblings,[45,46] but the relapse rate is only minimally affected by T-cell depletion.[16,47] Approximately one third of AML or myelodysplasia (MDS) patients respond to DLI, but these remissions are generally transient, and patients typically recur within one year.[3,5,48,49] Approximately one third of patients with multiple myeloma[50,51] also respond to DLI, but like AML, these responses are usually transient.

There is relatively little data to assess the responsiveness of HD to GVM effects. Few allogeneic transplants have been carried out in HD, and they have typically involved patients with advanced disease. A registry analysis could not detect a GVM effect in HD.[52] Recently, however, pilot studies have described responses to non-ablative transplants (Anderlini *et al.*, in press).[53]

Of the major leukemias, acute lymphoid leukemia (ALL) appears to be least affected by GVM,[16,17,46] possibly because of the lack of costimulatory molecules and limited capacity of the leukemic lymphoblasts to stimulate an effective immune response.[54,55] In addition, the rapid rate of proliferation of

ALL may outpace a developing immune response. Similar considerations apply to high-grade lymphomas.

A major question is whether GVM effects occur against solid tumors. Pilot studies in breast cancer have reported anti-tumor responses in patients with GVHD suggesting a GVM effect.[56,57] Limited data suggests GVM effects also occur against renal cell cancer and potentially other malignancies.[58–60] Further studies are required to determine whether the effects of a GVM response are clinically meaningful enough in solid tumors to justify the added morbidity associated with allogeneic transplantation.

Preliminary results with non-ablative preparative regimens

Purine analogs (fludarabine or cladribine) have activity against a wide range of hematologic malignancies and are sufficiently immunosuppressive to allow engraftment of HLA compatible hematopoietic progenitor cells. Giralt *et al.* initially evaluated the use of standard-dose purine analog-based chemotherapy as a non-ablative preparative regimen in patients with advanced myeloid leukemias.[61] Fludarabine 30 mg/m^2 for 4 days, cytarabine 1 g/m^2 for 4 days and idarubicin 12 mg/m^2 for 3 days was successful in achieving engraftment in patients with myeloid leukemias with a matched sibling donor; extended remissions were observed in over 50% of patients with CML[10] or recurrent chemotherapy-sensitive AML.[61] The combination of fludarabine 25–30 mg/m^2 for 4–5 days + cyclophosphamide at doses $\geq$ 1 g/m^2 for 2 days has been effective in inducing engraftment in a range of malignancies.[11,59,62]

In a follow up to the initial study 36 patients aged 55–75 years with AML, MDS or CML were treated with fludarabine, cytarabine and idarubicin followed by allogeneic hematologic transplantation from an HLA-matched or 1 antigen-mismatched sibling donor.[63] Patients with residual or recurrent disease received DLI or a second non-ablative transplant. Ninety-one percent of patients engrafted; 88% achieved complete remission. Treatment related mortality was $20 \pm 7\%$. Acute GVHD grade II–IV developed in $32 \pm 9\%$ of patients, and $52 \pm 14\%$ developed chronic GVHD. Fourteen patients are alive with a median follow-up of 11.5 months (range 4–40 months); 13 patients are currently disease-free. The projected survival of patients who were in remission or had < 10% bone marrow blasts at the time of transplant is $71 \pm 11\%$ and $59 \pm 14\%$ at 1 and 2 years, respectively. The disease-free survival is $65 \pm 12\%$ and $52 \pm 15\%$ at 1 and 2 years. The outcome of patients with refractory disease at transplant is poor; < 10% remained in remission at one year. A favorable outcome is expected if the disease is in remission at the time of transplant. These data indicate that NST is feasible in elderly patients and is associated with acceptable toxicity and GVHD rates.

Giralt *et al.* reported a second study combining melphalan (180 mg/m^2) and fludarabine (125 mg/m^2) for the treatment of advanced acute leukemia; this regimen was sufficiently immunosuppressive to allow engraftment in unrelated or 1 antigen-mismatched related transplants. Disease usually recurred in patients who were in refractory relapse at the time of transplant, but 56% of patients with chemotherapy-sensitive disease remained in continuous remission beyond one year.[63]

Slavin and coworkers reported use of a reduced toxicity preparative regimen consisting of busulfan 8 mg/kg, fludarabine and antithymocyte globulin.[12] Although less intensive and less toxic than commonly used ablative preparative regimens, this regimen produces marked myelosuppression and has not been administered without hematopoietic transplantation.

Another innovative approach involves treatment with low-dose total body irradiation (2 Gy) with or without fludarabine. This regimen is minimally myelosuppressive, but allows engraftment in a high fraction of patients.[64,65] Patients achieve initial mixed chimerism and subsequent GVM effects are seen;[66] remissions have been reported in patients with a range of hematologic malignancies. Other lower dose or non-ablative regimens have been proposed.[67–69]

Khouri *et al.* treated 15 patients with advanced CLL or transformed lymphoma using a non-myeloablative regimen of fludarabine + cyclophosphamide or fludarabine, cytarabine + cisplatin.[11] All patients had failed to respond to or had recurred after primary chemotherapy. Eleven of 15 patients had durable engraftment, with 50–100% donor cells at one month post-transplant, typically converting to 100% over the next two months, either spontaneously or after DLI. Hematopoietic recovery was prompt and no non-hematologic toxicities > grade II occurred. All 11 patients with engraftment responded and eight have achieved complete remission. Maximal responses were slow to develop and gradually occurred over a one-year period. The patients failing to engraft recovered hematopoiesis promptly and experienced no serious adverse effects.

Extending these studies to low-grade lymphoma, eleven patients received fludarabine 25 mg/m^2 for 5 days with cyclophosphamide 1 g/m^2 on day 4 and 5, followed by allogeneic stem cell transplantation. All patients achieved engraftment and complete remission with no treatment related mortality.[70] The procedure was associated with minimal toxicity. This compares favorably to results seen with high-dose cyclophosphamide–total body irradiation regimens in which treatment-related mortality rates typically exceed 30%.[71]

Allogeneic bone marrow transplantation is associated with a high risk of treatment related mortality in multiple myeloma – up to 70% in some series.[72,73] Using NST may reduce this morbidity while harnessing a GVM effect. Giralt *et al.* studied the use of melphalan (140 mg/m^2) and fludarabine (30 mg/m^2 for 4 days) in patients with advanced myeloma; 7 of 13 patients achieved complete remission.[74] This promising approach requires further study.

Indications for NST

Non-ablative regimens are only useful in malignancies susceptible to GVM effects. NST has generally been unsuccessful in patients with active, aggressive malignancies such as refractory acute leukemias.[61] In these patients, the malignancy may recur rapidly after a non-ablative regimen, outpacing generation of a GVM effect. Non-ablative regimens may be useful, however, for consolidation of remission in AML patients at high risk of relapse. Indolent malignancies which are not immediately life threatening appear to be the best candidates for this strategy; responses developing over several months can be effective in patients with chronic phase CML or low-grade lymphoid malignancies. Complete responses may occur in these diseases even in patients with extensive disease.

The optimal intensity of the preparative regimen depends on several factors including the disease status and aggressiveness of the patient's malignancy, immunocompetence of the recipient, and histocompatibility differences between the donor and recipient. Immunocompromised patients, such as those with advanced CLL, require less intensive immunosuppressive therapy to achieve engraftment than a fully immunocompetent recipient. Non-ablative regimens have generally been studied in patients with an HLA-identical sibling donor. Greater immunosuppression will be required for engraftment of HLA-non-identical or unrelated transplants.

The optimal post-transplant immunosuppressive therapy is also uncertain. Acute GVHD does occur with these non-ablative regimens but has been relatively mild and easily controlled. Immunosuppressive therapy given early post-transplant to prevent GVHD probably inhibits GVL.[75,76] The indications for DLI need to be clarified. Effective strategies to separate GVHD from GVL are critical for the success of NST.

Non-ablative hematopoietic transplants may become a platform for administration of cellular immunotherapy. An ideal cellular therapy would consist of malignancy-specific effectors devoid of graft-versus-host activity. Falkenburg *et al*. reported a single patient with CML who relapsed after allogeneic transplantation and failed to respond to DLI.[77] This patient was treated with an infusion of T-cell lines raised against the leukemia and achieved a complete response without development of GVHD. The technology for development of therapeutic T-cell clones is demanding, and this approach is not sufficiently developed to allow for large-scale clinical trials. For hematopoietic malignancies, cytotoxic T-lymphocytes specific for minor histocompatibility antigens limited to myeloid or lymphoid cells could be used.[78] Alternatively T-cells reactive against overexpressed malignancy-related antigens could be selected, expanded and parenterally administered as adoptive cellular therapy.[79]

In summary

The use of relatively non-toxic, non-myeloablative preparative regimens can result in engraftment and the generation of GVM effects. This approach is potentially curative for susceptible malignancies without the need for high-dose chemotherapy. This reduces the risks of treatment-related morbidity and allows the use of allotransplantation in older patients and in those with comorbidities which preclude high-dose chemoradiotherapy.

The indications for a non-myeloablative versus a high-dose ablative preparative regimen remain to be clearly defined. The benefit of reduced toxicity with non-ablative regimens may be offset by the loss of cytoreduction induced by high-dose chemotherapy. At present, young patients with myeloid malignancies in good physical condition have established benefits with high-dose ablative transplant regimens, and non-ablative regimens might best be studied in patients aged > 55 years or those with major medical comorbidities. The role of allogeneic hematopoietic transplantation is less established in the indolent lymphoid malignancies and the encouraging data reported above supports further testing in patients of all ages. Patients should be treated within the context of clinical trials designed to address outstanding issues. Ultimately, controlled trials are needed to define the relative efficacy of non-ablative versus ablative hematopoietic transplants and non-ablative transplants versus alternative forms of transplantation as well as standard (non-transplant) treatments.

References

1.   Thomas ED. Bone marrow transplantation for malignant disease. *J Clin Oncol* 1983; 1: 517.

2.   Thomas ED. The role of bone marrow transplantation for eradication of malignant disease. *Cancer* 1969; 10: 1963–9.

3.   Collins RH Jr, Shpilberg O, Drobyski WR, Porter DL, Giralt S, Champlin R, Goodman SA, Wolff SN, Hu W, Verfaillie C, List A, Dalton W, Ognoskie N, Chetrit A, Antin JH, Nemunaitis J. Donor leukocyte infusions in 140 patients with relapsed malignancy after allogeneic bone marrow transplantation. *J Clin Oncol* 1997; 15: 433–44.

4.   Giralt SA, Champlin RE. Leukemia relapse after allogeneic bone marrow transplantation: A review. *Blood* 1994; 84: 3603–12.

5.   Kolb HJ, Schattenberg A, Goldman JM, Hertenstein B, Jacobsen N, Arcese W, Ljungman P, Ferrant A, Verdonck L, Niederwieser D, Van Rhee F, Mittermueller J, de Witte T, Holler E, Ansari H. Graft-vs-leukemia effect of donor lymphocyte transfusions in marrow grafted patients. *Blood* 1995; 86: 2041–50.

6.   Hoffmann T, Theobald M, Bunjes D, Weiss M, Heimpel H, Heit W. Frequency of bone marrow T cells responding to HLA-identical non-leukemic and leukemic stimulator cells. *Bone Marrow Transpl* 1993; 12: 1–8.

7.   Keil F, Haas OA, Fritsch G, Kalhs P, Lechner K, Mannhalter C, Reiter E, Niederwieser D, Hoecker P, Greinix HT. Donor leukocyte infusion for leukemic relapse after allogeneic marrow transplantation: Lack of residual donor hematopoiesis predicts aplasia. *Blood* 1997; 89: 3113–17.

8.   Van Rhee F, Lin F, Cullis JO, Spencer A, Cross NCP, Chase A, Garicochea B, Bungey J, Barrett J, Goldman JM. Relapse of chronic myeloid leukemia after allogeneic bone marrow transplant: The case for giving donor leukocyte transfusions before the onset of hematologic relapse. *Blood* 1994; 83: 3377–83.

9.   Ribas A, Bui LA, Butterfield LH, Vollmer CM, Jilani SM, Dissette VB, Glaspy JA, McBride WH, Economou JS. Antitumor protection using murine dendritic cells pulsed with acid-eluted peptides from *in vivo* grown tumors of different immunogenicities. *Anticancer Res* 1999; 19: 1165–70.

10. Giralt S, Gajewski J, Khouri I, Korbling M, Claxton D, Mehra R, Przepiorka D, Andersson B, Talpaz M, Kantarjian H, Champlin R. Induction of graft-versus-leukemia as primary treatment of chronic myelogenous leukemia. *Blood* 1997; 90 (Suppl 1): 1857a.

11. Khouri I, Keating M, Korbling M, Przepiorka D, Anderlini P, O'Brien S, Von Wolff B, Giralt S, Gajewski JG, Mehra R, Ippoliti C, Claxton D, Champlin RE. Transplant lite: induction of graft-versus-leukemia using fludarabine-based nonablative chemotherapy and allogeneic blood progenitor cell transplantation as treatment for lymphoid malignancies. *J Clin Oncol* 1998; 16: 2817–24.

12. Slavin S, Nagler A, Naparstek E, Kapelushnik Y, Aker M, Cividalli G, Varadi G, Kirschbaum M, Ackerstein A, Samuel S, Amar A, Brautbar C, Ben-Tal O, Eldor A, Or R. Non-myeloablative stem cell transplantation and cell therapy as an alternative to conventional bone marrow transplantation with lethal cytoreduction for the treatment of malignant and nonmalignant hematologic diseases. *Blood* 1998; 91: 756–63.

13. Storb R, Yu C, Wagner JL, Deeg HJ, Nash RA, Kiem HP, Leisenring W, Shulman H. Stable mixed hematopoietic chimerism in DLA-identical littermate dogs given sublethal total body irradiation before and pharmacological immunosuppression after marrow transplantation. *Blood* 1997; 89: 3048–54.

14. Antin JH, Ferrara JLM. Cytokine dysregulation and acute graft-versus-host disease. *Blood* 1992; 80: 2964–8.

15. Hill GR, Crawford JM, Cooke KR, Brinson YS, Pan LY, Ferrara JLM. Total body irradiation and acute graft-versus-host disease: The role of gastrointestinal damage and inflammatory cytokines. *Blood* 1997; 90: 3204–13.

16. Marmont AM, Horowitz MM, Gale RP, Sobocinski K, Ash RC, van Bekkum DW, Champlin RE, Dicke KA, Goldman JM, Good RA, Herzig RH, Hong R, Masaoka T, Rimm AA, Ringdén O, Speck B, Weiner RS, Bortin MM. T-cell depletion of HLA-identical transplants in leukemia. *Blood* 1991; 78: 2120–30.

17. Horowitz MM, Gale RP, Sondel PM, Goldman JM, Kersey J, Kolb H-J, Rimm AA, Ringdén O, Rozman C, Speck B, Truitt RL, Zwaan FE, Bortin MM. Graft-versus-leukemia reactions after bone marrow transplantation. *Blood* 1990; 75: 555–62.

18. Apperley JF, Jones L, Hale G, Waldmann H, Hows J, Rombos Y, Tsatalas C, Marcus RE, Goolden AWG, Gordon-Smith EC, Catovsky D, Galton DAG, Goldman JM. Bone marrow transplantation for patients with chronic myeloid leukaemia: T-cell depletion with Campath-1 reduces the incidence of graft-versus-host disease but may increase the risk of leukaemic relapse. *Bone Marrow Transpl* 1986; 1: 53–68

19. Goldman JM, Gale RP, Bortin MM, Biggs JC, Champlin RE, Gluckman E, Hoffmann RG, Horowitz MM, Marmont AM, McGlave PB, Messner HA, Rimm AA, Rozman C, Speck B, Tura S, Weiner RS. Bone marrow transplantation for chronic myelogenous leukemia in chronic phase: increased risk of relapse associated with T-cell depletion. *Ann Intern Med* 1988; 108: 806–14.

20. Mackinnon S, Barnett L, Heller G, O'Reilly RJ. Minimal residual disease is more common in patients who have mixed T-cell chimerism after bone marrow transplantation for chronic myelogenous leukemia. *Blood* 1994; 83: 3409–16.

21. Offit K, Burns JP, Cunningham I, Jhanwar SC, Black P, Kernan NA, O'Reilly RJ, Chaganti RSK. Cytogenetic analysis of chimerism and leukemia relapse in chronic myelogenous leukemia patients after T cell-depleted bone marrow transplantation. *Blood* 1990; 75: 1346–55.

22. Apperley JF, Rassool F, Parreira A, Geary CG, Harrison C, Stansfield D, Goldman JM. Philadelphia-positive metaphases in the marrow after bone marrow transplantation for chronic granulocytic leukemia. *Am J Hematol* 1986; 22: 199–204.

23. Radich JP, Gehly G, Gooley T, Bryant E, Clift RA, Collins S, Edmands S, Kirk J, Lee A, Kessler P, Schoch G, Buckner CD, Sullivan KM, Appelbaum FR, Thomas ED. Polymerase chain reaction detection of the BCR-ABL fusion transcript after allogeneic marrow transplantation for chronic myeloid leukemia: Results and implications in 346 patients. *Blood* 1995; 85: 2632–38.

24. Hughes TP, Morgan GJ, Martiat P, Goldman JM. Detection of residual leukemia after bone marrow transplant for chronic myeloid leukemia: Role of polymerase chain reaction in predicting relapse. *Blood* 1991; 77: 874–8.

25. Pichert G, Alyea EP, Soiffer RJ, Roy D-C, Ritz J. Persistence of myeloid progenitor cells expressing BCR-ABL mRNA after allogeneic bone marrow transplantation for chronic myelogenous leukemia. *Blood* 1994; 84: 2109–14.

26. DeLage R, Soiffer RJ, Dear K, Ritz J. Clinical significance of bcr-abl gene rearrangement detected by polymerase chain reaction after allogeneic bone marrow transplantation in chronic myelogenous leukemia. *Blood* 1991; 78: 2759–67.

27. Lee M, Khouri I, Champlin R, Kantarjian H, Talpaz M, Trujillo J, Freireich E, Deisseroth A, Stass S. Detection of minimal residual disease by polymerase chain reaction of bcr/abl transcripts in chronic myelogenous leukaemia following allogeneic bone marrow transplantation. *Br J Haematol* 1992; 82: 708–14.

28. Pichert G, Ritz J. Clinical significance of bcr-abl gene rearrangement detected by the polymerase chain reaction after allogeneic bone marrow transplantation in chronic myelogenous leukemia. *Leuk Lymphoma* 1993; 10: 1–8.

29. Sawyers CL, Timson L, Kawasaki ES, Clark SS, Witte ON, Champlin R. Molecular relapse in chronic myelogenous leukemia patients after bone marrow transplantation detected by polymerase chain reaction. *Proc Natl Acad Sci USA* 1990; 87: 563–7.

30. Rapanotti MC, Arcese W, Buffolino S, Iori AP, Mengarelli A, De Cuia MR, Cardillo A, Cimino G. Sequential molecular monitoring of chimerism in chronic myeloid leukemia patients receiving donor lymphocyte transfusion for relapse after bone marrow transplantation. *Bone Marrow Transpl* 1997; 19: 703–07.

31. Cullis JO, Jiang YZ, Schwarer AP, Hughes TP, Barrett AJ, Goldman JM. Donor leukocyte infusions for chronic myeloid leukemia in relapse after allogeneic bone marrow transplantation. *Blood* 1992; 79: 1379–81.

32. Raanani P, Dazzi F, Sohal J, Szydlo RM, Van Rhee F, Reiter A, Lin F, Goldman JM, Cross NCP. The rate and kinetics of molecular response to donor leucocyte transfusions in chronic myeloid leukaemia patients treated for relapse after allogeneic bone marrow transplantation. *Br J Haematol* 1997; 99: 945–50.

33. Antin JH. Graft-versus-leukemia: No longer an epiphenomenon. *Blood* 1993; 82: 2273–77.

34. Drobyski WR, Keever CA, Roth MS, Koethe S, Hanson G, McFadden P, Gottschall JL, Ash RC, Van Tuinen P, Horowitz MM, Flomenberg N. Salvage immunotherapy using donor leukocyte infusions as treatment for relapsed chronic myelogenous leukemia after allogeneic bone marrow transplantation: Efficacy and toxicity of a defined T-cell dose. *Blood* 1993; 82: 2310–18.

35. Bacigalupo A, Soracco M, Vassallo F, Abate M, Van Lint MT, Gualandi F, Lamparelli T, Occhini D, Mordini N, Bregante S, Figari O, Benvenuto F, Sessarego M, Fugazza G, Carlier P, Valbonesi M. Donor lymphocyte infusions (DLI) in patients with chronic myeloid leukemia following allogeneic bone marrow transplantation. *Bone Marrow Transpl* 1997; 19: 927–32.

36. Dazzi F, Szydlo RM, Goldman JM. Donor lymphocyte infusions for relapse of chronic myeloid leukemia after allogeneic stem cell transplant: Where we now stand. *Exp Hematol* 1999; 27: 1477–86.

37. Rondón G, Giralt S, Huh Y, Khouri I, Andersson B, Andreeff M, Champlin R. Graft-versus-leukemia effect after allogeneic bone marrow transplantation for chronic lymphocytic leukemia. *Bone Marrow Transpl* 1996; 18: 669–72.

38. Van Besien KW, De Lima M, Giralt SA, Moore DF, Jr., Khouri IF, Rondón G, Mehra R, Andersson BS, Dyer C, Cleary K, Przepiorka D, Gajewski JL, Champlin RE. Management of lymphoma recurrence after allogeneic transplantation: The relevance of graft-versus-lymphoma effect. *Bone Marrow Transpl* 1997; 19: 977–82.

39. Khouri I, Keating MJ, Przepiorka D, O'Brien S, Giralt S, Korbling M, Champlin R. Engraftment and induction of GVL with fludarabine-based non-ablative preparative regimen in patients with chronic lymphocytic leukemia. *Blood* 1996; 88 (Suppl. 1): 301a.

40. Van Besien K, Sobocinski K, Rowlings PA, Murphy SC, Armitage JO, Bishop MR, Chaekal OK, Gale RP, Klein JP, Lazarus HM, McCarthy PL Jr, Raemaekers JMM, Reiffers J, Phillips GL, Schattenberg AVMB, Verdonck LF, Vose JM, Horowitz MM. Allogeneic bone marrow transplantation for low-grade lymphoma. *Blood* 1998; 92: 1832–6.

41. Khouri IF, Przepiorka D, Van Besien K, O'Brien S, Palmer JL, Lerner S, Mehra RC, Vriesendorp HM, Andersson BS, Giralt S, Körbling M, Keating MJ, Champlin RE. Allogeneic blood or marrow transplantation for chronic lymphocytic leukaemia: Timing of transplantation and potential effect of fludarabine on acute graft-versus-host disease. *Br J Haematol* 1997; 97: 466–73.

42. Michallet M, Archimbaud E, Bandini G, Rowlings PA, Deeg HJ, Gahrton G, Montserrat E, Rozman C, Gratwohl A, Gale RP. HLA-identical sibling bone marrow transplantation in younger patients with chronic lymphocytic leukemia. *Ann Intern Med* 1996; 124: 311–15.

43. Khouri I, Lee MS, Palmer L, Giralt S, McLaughlin P, Korbling M, Romaguera J, Donato M, Younes A, Ueno N, Gajewski J, Cabanillas F, Champlin R. Transplant-lite using fludarabine–cyclophosphamide and allogeneic stem cell transplant for low grade lymphoma. *Blood* 1999; 94 (Suppl. 1): 1553a.

43. Khouri I, Keating M, Korbling M, Przepiorka D, Anderlini P, O'Brien S, Von Wolff B, Giralt S, Gajewski JG, Mehra R, Ippoliti C, Claxton D, Champlin RE. Transplant lite: induction of graft-versus-leukemia using fludarabine-based nonablative chemotherpy and allogeneic blood progenitor cell transplantation as treatment for lymphoid malignancies. *J Clin Oncol* 1998; 16: 2817–24.

45. Gale RP, Champlin RE. How does bone marrow transplantation cure leukemia? *Lancet* 1984; 2: 28–30.

46. Gale RP, Horowitz MM, Ash RC, Champlin RE, Goldman JM, Rimm AA, Ringdén O, Stone JAV, Bortin MM. Identical-twin bone marrow transplants for leukemia. *Ann Intern Med* 1994; 120: 646–52.

47. Papadopoulos EB, Carabasi MH, Castro-Malaspina H, Childs BH, Mackinnon S, Boulad F, Gillio AP, Kernan NA, Small TN, Szabolcs P, Taylor J, Yahalom J, Collins NH, Bleau SA, Black PM, Heller G, O'Reilly RJ, Young JW. T-cell-depleted allogeneic bone marrow transplantation as postremission therapy for acute myelogenous leukemia: Freedom from relapse in the absence of graft-versus-host disease. *Blood* 1998; 91: 1083–90.

48. Porter DL, Roth MS, Lee SJ, McGarigle C, Ferrara JLM, Antin JH. Adoptive immunotherapy with donor mononuclear cell infusions to treat relapse of acute leukemia or myelodysplasia after allogeneic bone marrow transplantation. *Bone Marrow Transpl* 1996; 18: 975–80.

49. Okumura H, Takamatsu H, Yoshida T. Donor leucocyte transfusions for relapse in myelodysplastic syndrome after allogeneic bone marrow transplantation. *Br J Haematol* 1996; 93: 386–8.

50. Lokhorst HM, Schattenberg A, Cornelissen JJ, Thomas LLM, Verdonck LF. Donor leukocyte infusions are effective in relapsed multiple myeloma after allogeneic bone marrow transplantation. *Blood* 1997; 90: 4206–11.

51. Tricot G, Vesole DH, Jagannath S, Hilton J, Munshi N, Barlogie B. Graft-versus-myeloma effect: Proof of principle. *Blood* 1996; 87: 1196–8.

52. Gajewski JL, Phillips GL, Sobocinski KA, Armitage JO, Gale RP, Champlin RE, Herzig RH, Hurd DD, Jagannath S, Klein JP, Lazarus HM, McCarthy PL Jr, Pavlovsky S, Petersen FB, Rowlings PA, Russell JA, Silver SM, Vose JM, Wiernik PH, Bortin MM, Horowitz MM. Bone marrow transplants from HLA-identical siblings in advanced Hodgkin's disease. *J Clin Oncol* 1996; 14: 572–8.

53. Carella AM, Champlin R, Slavin S, McSweeney P, Storb R. Mini-allografts: ongoing trials in humans. *Bone Marrow Transpl* 2000; 25: 345–50.

54. Cardoso AA, Seamon MJ, Afonso HM, Ghia P, Boussiotis VA, Freeman GJ, Gribben JG, Sallan SE, Nadler LM. *Ex vivo* generation of human anti-pre-B leukemia-specific autologous cytolytic T cells. *Blood* 1997; 90: 549–61.

55. Brenner M, Porcelli S. Antigen presentation: A balanced diet. *Science* 1997; 277: 332.

56. Ueno NT, Rondón G, Mirza NQ, Geisler DK, Anderlini P, Giralt SA, Andersson BS, Claxton DF, Gajewski JL, Khouri IF, Körbling M, Mehra RC, Przepiorka D, Rahman Z, Samuels BI, Van Besien K, Hortobagyi GN, Champlin RE. Allogeneic peripheral-blood progenitor-cell transplantation for poor-risk patients with metastatic breast cancer. *J Clin Oncol* 1998; 16: 986–93.

57. Eibl B, Schwaighofer H, Nachbaur D, Marth C, Gächter A, Knapp R, Böck G, Gassner C, Schiller L, Petersen F, Niederwieser D. Evidence for a graft-versus-tumor effect in a patient treated with marrow ablative chemotherapy and allogeneic bone marrow transplantation for breast cancer. *Blood* 1996; 88: 1501–08.

58. Childs RW, Clave E, Tisdale J, Plante M, Hensel N, Barrett J. Successful treatment of metastatic renal cell carcinoma with a nonmyeloablative allogeneic peripheral-blood progenitor-cell transplant: Evidence for a graft-versus-tumor effect. *J Clin Oncol* 1999; 17: 2044–9.

59. Childs R, Clave E, Contentin N, Jayasekera D, Hensel N, Leitman S, Read EJ, Carter C, Bahceci E, Young NS, Barrett AJ. Engraftment kinetics after nonmyeloablative allogeneic peripheral blood stem cell transplantation: Full donor T-cell chimerism precedes alloimmune responses. *Blood* 1999; 94: 3234–41.

60. Ueno NT, Rondón G, Mirza NQ, Geisler DK, Anderlini P, Giralt SA, Andersson BS, Claxton DF, Gajewski JL, Khouri IF, Körbling M, Mehra RC, Przepiorka D, Rahman Z, Samuels BI, Van Besien K, Hortobagyi GN, Champlin RE. Allogeneic peripheral-blood progenitor-cell transplantation for poor-risk patients with metastatic breast cancer. *J Clin Oncol* 1998; 16: 986–93.

61. Giralt S, Estey E, Albitar M, Van Besien K, Rondon G, Anderlini P, O'Brien S, Khouri I, Gajewski J, Mehra R, Claxton D, Andersson B, Beran M, Przepiorka D, Koller C, Kornblau S, Körbling M, Keating M, Kantarjian H, Champlin R. Engraftment of allogeneic hematopoietic progenitor cells with purine analog-containing chemotherapy: Harnessing graft-versus-leukemia without myeloablative therapy. *Blood* 1997; 89: 4531–6.

62. Carella AM, Lerma E, Dejana A, Corsetti MT, Celesti L, Bruni R, Benvenuto F, Figari O, Parodi C, Carlier P, Florio G, Lercari G, Valbonesi M, Casarino L, De Stefano F, Geniram A, Venturino M, Tedeschi L, Palmieri G, Piaggio G, Podestà M, Frassoni F, Van Lint MT, Marmont AM. Engraftment of HLA-matched sibling hematopoietic stem cells after immunosuppressive conditioning regimen in patients with hematologic neoplasias. *Haematologica* 1998; 83: 904–09.

63. Giralt S, Cohen A, Mehra R, Gajewski J, Andersson B, Przepiorka D, Khouri I, Korbling M, Davis M, Van Besien K, Ippoliti C, Bruton J, Anderlini P, Ueno N, Champlin R. Preliminary results of fludarabine/melphalan or 2CDA/melphalan as preparative regimens for allogeneic progenitor cell transplantation in poor candidates for conventional myeloablative conditioning. *Blood* 1997; 90: (Suppl. 1): 1853a.

64. Storb R, Yu C, Sandmaier B, McSweeney P, Georges G, Nash R, Woolfrey A. Mixed hematopoietic chimerism after hematopoietic stem cell allografts. *Transpl Proc* 1999; 31: 677–8.

65. Storb R, Yu C, Sandmaier BM, McSweeney PA, Georges G, Nash RA, Woolfrey A. Mixed hematopoietic chimerism after marrow allografts – Transplantation in the ambulatory care setting. *Ann NY Acad Sci* 1999; 872: 372–6.

66. McSweeney P, Niederwieser D, Shizuru J, Molina A, Wagner J, Minor S, Radich J, Chauncey T, Hegenhart U, Maloney D, Nash R, Sandmaier B, Blume K, Storb R. Outpatient allografting with minimally myelosuppressive immunosuppressive conditioning of low-dose TBI and postgrafting cyclosporine and mycophenolate mofetil. *Blood* 1999; 94 (Suppl. 1): 393a.

67. Kelemen E, Massszi T, Reményi P, Barta A, Pálóczi K. Reduction in the frequency of transplant-related complications in patients with chronic myeloid leukemia undergoing BMT preconditioned with a new, non-myeloablative drug combination. *Bone Marrow Transpl* 1998; 21: 747–9.

68. Sykes M, Preffer F, McAfee S, Saidman SL, Weymouth D, Andrews DM, Colby C, Sackstein R, Sachs DH, Spitzer TR. Mixed lymphohaemopoietic chimerism and graft-versus-lymphoma effects after non-myeloablative therapy and HLA-mismatched bone-marrow transplantation. *Lancet* 1999; 353: 1755–9.

69. Khoury H, Adkins D, Pence H, Vij R, Brown R, Goodnough T, Wetervelt P, Lin S, DiPersio J. Low transplant related acute complications in patients with CML undergoing allogeneic stem cell transplantation with a low dose (550 cGy) total body irradiation conditioning regimen. *Blood* 1999; 94 (Suppl. 1): 393a.

70. Khouri I, Lee MS, Palmer L, Giralt S, McLaughlin P, Korbling M, Romeguera J, Donato M, Younes A, Ueno N, Gajewski J, Cabanillas F, Champlin R. Transplant-lite using fludarabine–cyclophosphamide and allogeneic stem cell transplantation for low grade lymphoma. *Blood* 1999; 94: 1553a.

71. Van Besien K, Sobocinski K, Rowlings PA, Murphy SC, Armitage JO, Bishop MR, Chaekal OK, Gale RP, Klein JP, Lazarus HM, McCarthy PL, Jr, Raemaekers JMM, Reiffers J, Phillips GL, Schattenberg AVMB, Verdonck LF, Vose JM, Horowitz MM. Allogeneic bone marrow transplantation for low-grade lymphoma. *Blood* 1998; 92: 1832–6.

72. Bensinger WI, Buckner CD, Anasetti C, Clift R, Storb R, Barnett T, Chauncey T, Shulman H, Appelbaum FR. Allogeneic marrow transplantation for multiple myeloma: An analysis of risk factors on outcome. *Blood* 1996; 88: 2787–93.

73. Gahrton G, Tura S, Ljungman P, Bladé J, Brandt L, Cavo M, Façon T, Gratwohl A, Hagenbeek A, Jacobs P, De Laurenzi A, Van Lint M, Michallet M, Nikoskelainen J, Reiffers J, Samson D, Verdonck L, de Witte T, Volin L. Prognostic factors in allogeneic bone marrow transplantation for multiple myeloma. *J Clin Oncol* 1995; 13: 1312–22.

74. Bertucci F, Viens P, Gravis G, Blaise D, Faucher C, Oziel-Taoeb S, Bardou VJ, Jacquemier J, Delpero JR, Maraninchi D. High-dose chemotherapy with hematopoietic stem cell support in patients with advanced epithelial ovarian cancer: Analysis of 67 patients treated in a single institution. *Anticancer Res* 1999; 19: 1455–61.

75. Bacigalupo A, Vitale V, Corvò R, Barra S, Lamparelli T, Gualandi F, Mordini N, Berisso G, Bregante S, Raiola AM, Van Lint MT, Frassoni F. The combined effect of total body irradiation (TBI) and cyclosporin A (CyA) on the risk of relapse in patients with acute myeloid leukaemia undergoing allogeneic bone marrow transplantation. *Br J Haematol* 2000; 108: 99–104.

76. Locatelli F, Zecca M, Rondelli R, Bonetti F, Dini G, Prete A, Messina C, Uderzo C, Ripaldi M, Porta F, Giorgiani G, Giraldi E, Pession A. Graft versus host disease prophylaxis with low-dose cyclosporine-A reduces the risk of relapse in children with acute leukemia given HLA-identical sibling bone marrow transplantation: results of a randomized trial. *Blood* 2000; 95: 1572–9.

77. Smit WM, Rijnbeek M, Van Bergen CAM, Willemze R, Falkenburg JHF: Generation of leukemia-reactive cytotoxic T lymphocytes from HLA- identical donors of patients with chronic myeloid leukemia using modifications of a limiting dilution assay. *Bone Marrow Transpl* 1998; 21: 553–60.

78. Mutis T, Verdijk R, Schrama E, Esendam B, Brand A, Goulmy E. Feasibility of immunotherapy of relapsed leukemia with *ex vivo*-generated cytotoxic T lymphocytes specific for hematopoietic system-restricted minor histocompatibility antigens. *Blood* 1999; 93: 2336–41.

79. Molldrem JJ, Lee PP, Wang CQ, Champlin RE, Davis MM: A PR1-human leukocyte antigen-A2 tetramer can be used to isolate low-frequency cytotoxic T lymphocytes from healthy donors that selectively lyse chronic myelogenous leukemia. *Cancer Res* 1999; 59: 2675–81.

Non-myeloablative stem cell transplantation in myeloid leukemias – The M. D. Anderson Cancer Center experience

S Giralt

Introduction

The potency of the immune mediated graft-versus-leukemia (GVL) effect has been demonstrated by the ability of donor lymphocyte infusions (DLI) to reinduce remissions in patients who have relapsed after an allogeneic progenitor cell transplant. This effect is more pronounced in patients with chronic myelogenous leukemia (CML), but has also been observed in patients with acute myelogenous leukemia (AML), chronic lymphocytic leukemia (CLL), myeloma and other hematologic malignancies.[1–8] Thus, the GVL effect is sufficient to obtain long-term disease control without intense myeloablative therapy. Therefore less intensive conditioning regimens with sufficient immunosuppressive activity could allow for exploitation of a GVL effect without the toxicity of myeloablative therapy. These non-ablative therapies have now been applied to a variety of older or debilitated patients, or patients with benign disorders that are potentially curable with allogeneic transplantation.[9–12]

Non-myeloablative allogeneic progenitor cell transplantation (NST) is being explored with increasing frequency, as documented by the number of abstracts submitted for presentation to the meetings of the American Society of Hematology (ASH) and the number of patients reported to have undergone this procedure (Table 1). These reports have demonstrated the feasibility of NST, the ability of a variety of regimens to obtain engraftment of allogeneic progenitor cells, and the possibility of inducing long-term remissions in patients with a variety of disorders without the use of traditional myeloablative therapies.[12–23] However, the impact of these procedures on the long-term outcome of patients, as well as their place in current treatment strategies for the different disorders, remains to be defined.

Table 1. Clinical NST abstracts submitted to the annual ASH meeting between 1996 and 1999

Year	Number of abstracts	Number of patients
1996	3	17
1997	5	85
1998	8	141
1999	24	375

In this chapter current results from patients with AML, myelodysplastic syndromes (MDS), and CML who underwent NST transplantation at the M. D. Anderson Cancer Center (MDACC) between 1995 and 1999 will be discussed.

NST for AML or MDS

The primary eligibility criteria for the initial NST protocols at MDACC were
- availability of an HLA compatible donor and
- ineligibility for a conventional myeloablative protocol either because of age or medical condition.

Thirty one patients with AML and 4 patients with MDS have been treated. The median age was 61 years (range 27–74 years), and the majority of patients were refractory or beyond first salvage. Other patient characteristics as well as comorbidities are summarized in Table 2.

Patients received one of two preparative regimens depending on prior fludarabine exposure. Twenty patients who either had had no prior fludarabine exposure or had responded to prior fludarabine-based chemotherapy received fludarabine 30 mg/m^2 daily for 4 days in combination with cytarabine 2 g/m^2 4 hours after each fludarabine dose and idarubicin 12 mg/m^2 daily for 3 days (FLAG-ida). Eleven patients with prior fludarabine exposure received cladribine 12 mg/m^2 x 5 days by continuous infusion with cytarabine 1 g/m^2 daily.[24,25] All patients received fully matched or 1 antigen mismatched blood or bone marrow from a related donor 2 days after chemotherapy in conjunction with graft-versus-host disease (GVHD) prophylaxis. GVHD prophylaxis consisted of cyclosporine (CSA) or tacrolimus with either steroids or methotrexate.

Table 2. Characteristics of patients with AML/MDS undergoing NST at MDACC

Number of patients	35
Median age (range)	61 years (21–74 years)
Disease status at transplant	
CR1/first salvage	8/2
CR2/refractory or beyond first salvage	4/21
Median number prior therapies (range)	2 (1–5)
Median % blast pre-transplant (range)	
Bone marrow	3 (1–95)
Blood	0 (0–98)
Comorbidities	
Age > 55 years	30
Infection or PS > 2	7
Poor organ function	2
History CHF	8

CR1 = first complete remission, CR2 = second complete remission.

Neutrophil recovery occurred in 29 patients at a median of 13 days post-transplant (range 8–38 days) and 25 patients achieved platelet transfusion independence after a median of 17 days (range 8–78 days). Chimerism analysis by cytogenetic or restriction fraction length polymorphisms on day 30 revealed that 20 patients had between 80 and 100% donor cells, 1 patient had 40% donor cells and 2 patients had no evidence of donor cell engraftment. Two patients with > 90% engraftment had late autologous reconstitution by 3 months without evidence of relapse, all other patients in remission remained with > 90% donor cell engraftment.

Toxicity was minimal with only one treatment-related death. Acute GVHD grade ≥ II occurred in 6 patients, one patient died as a result of this complication. Grade ≥ II acute GVHD occurred in 4/9 recipients of mismatched bone marrow versus 2/24 patients receiving matched peripheral blood.

Complete remission (as defined by neutrophil recovery, platelet transfusion independence and < 5% bone marrow blasts) was obtained or continued in 24 patients. Relapse occurred in 13 of these patients at a median of 3.6 months (range 1.4–17.2 months). At 1 year the overall survival for the whole group is 47% and the disease-free survival is 34% (Figure 1). The most important prognostic factor for survival was disease status at the time of transplant. Patients who were in remission or untreated first relapse when they received their transplant had a better outcome than those with refractory disease (Figure 2). Death resulted from disease ($n = 15$), infection ($n = 3$), toxicity ($n = 1$), GVHD ($n = 1$) and graft failure ($n = 1$).

Salvage therapy for relapsing and non-responding patients consisted of immunosuppression withdrawal, G-CSF, salvage chemotherapy alone or with DLI. No patient achieved a long-term remission following salvage therapy. Only 3/5 patients who underwent a subsequent stem cell transplant after high-dose melphalan ($n = 3$), busulfan/cyclophosphamide ($n = 1$) or cladribine/ara-C ($n = 1$) achieved a second long-term remission.

NST for CML

CML would seem to be the ideal disease for exploration of NST, since it has a chronic course and is extremely sensitive to DLI, at least in the chronic phase.[2] In addition, CML patients are generally more immune-competent than patients with AML or MDS by virtue of their disease and having received less therapy. However, this could potentially result in a higher incidence of graft failure and/or subsequent autologous reconstitution.

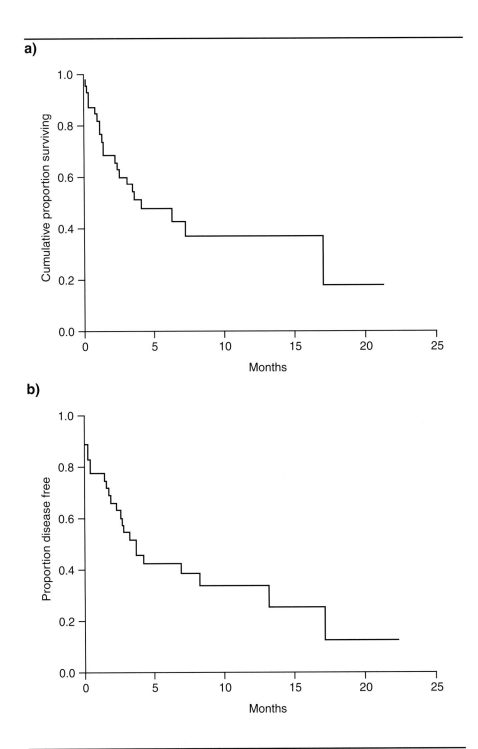

Figure 1. (a) Overall survival of AML/MDS patients undergoing NST with FLAG-ida or cladribine/ara-C at MDACC. (b) Disease-free survival of AML/MDS patients undergoing NST with FLAG-ida or cladribine/ara-C at MDACC.

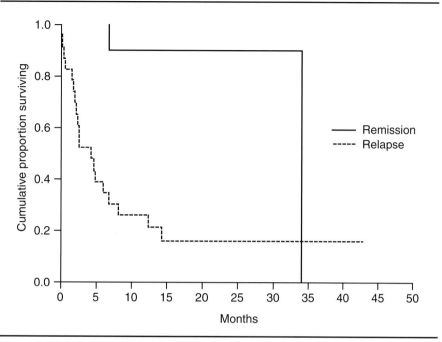

Figure 2. Survival of AML/MDS patients receiving NST according to disease status at transplantation.

Ten patients with CML have been treated with NST using the same preparative regimen (FLAG-ida) that was used for the AML/MDS patients. The median age of these patients was 57 years (range 42–71 years); all had failed prior interferon therapy, 5 were in late chronic phase and 5 were either in accelerated phase or blast crisis. Two patients received bone marrow from HLA identical unrelated donors, the remaining patients received peripheral blood stem cells from HLA-identical siblings. GVHD prophylaxis consisted primarily of CSA with or without methylprednisolone in 6 patients and tacrolimus/mini-methotrexate in 4 patients.

All patients had neutrophil recovery at a median of 13 days (range 10–31 days), and all became platelet transfusion independent at a median of 14 days (range 9–68 days). At day 30, 4 patients had 100% donor cell engraftment, 3 patients had between 15 and 80% donor cells and both recipients of unrelated donor cells had 100% autologous reconstitution without ever showing signs of donor cell engraftment. No patient died as a result of treatment-related toxicity, but 1 patient died from complications of acute GVHD.

At day 30 post-transplant, six patients had achieved complete or major cytogenetic remissions. Four of these patients subsequently relapsed – one responded

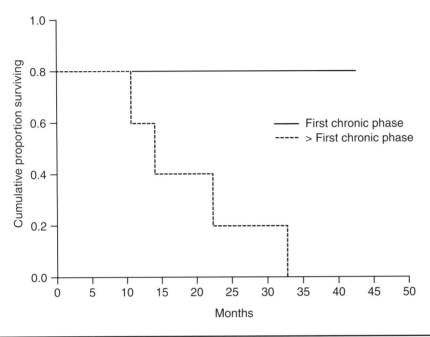

Figure 3. Overall survival of CML patients treated with NST at the MDACC.

to a DLI. Two of the 5 patients transplanted in chronic phase are alive in complete cytogenetic remission at 21 and 25 months post-transplant. None of the patients transplanted in transformed phase achieved long-term disease control (Figure 3).

Melphalan and purine analog combinations

The lack of engraftment of unrelated donor cells, and the poor results in patients with refractory disease prompted the search for reduced-intensity conditioning that, although not truly non-myeloablative, could still be tolerated by older or debilitated patients and provide sufficient leukemia control to allow time for a GVL effect to take place. The combination of melphalan with a purine analog was a rationale choice:

- melphalan is an alkylator agent with broad activity in a variety of hematologic malignancies
- melphalan is well tolerated as a single agent in debilitated patients because it induces few non-hematologic toxicities
- the combination of purine analogs and melphalan could be synergistic since purine analogs are known to inhibit some mechanisms of DNA repair.[26–28]

We treated 83 patients with melphalan/purine analog combinations between 1996 and 1999. Patient and treatment characteristics are summarized in Table 3. In brief, the median age was 54 years (range 22–70 years), 40 patients had AML or MDS and 33 patients had CML. Only 30 patients were transplanted in first chronic phase, first or subsequent remission or untreated first relapse, all other patients had advanced or refractory disease. Forty patients received cells from a fully-matched unrelated donor, while 43 patients received cells from fully-matched ($n = 37$) or 1-antigen-mismatched ($n = 6$) related donors. The median time to transplant was 16 months (range 1–220 months), the median number of prior therapies was 2, with 18 patients having failed a prior high-dose chemotherapy program. Seventy-seven patients were conditioned with fludarabine 25 mg/m^2 daily for 5 days and melphalan 180 mg/m^2 ($n = 65$) or 140 mg/m^2 ($n = 12$) (FM), while 6 patients received cladribine 12 mg/m^2

Table 3. Characteristics of patients receiving purine analog/melphalan combinations

Median age (range)	54 years (22–70 years)
Diagnosis	
AML	37
MDS	13
CML	33
Status at transplant	
Early leukemia (CR1/CP1)	1/8
Untreated first salvage	14
Remission ≥ 2	7
Transformed CML	25
Refractory or beyond first relapse	28
Comorbid conditions	
Age > 50 years	51
Muga < 50%	4
PFTs < 50%	5
GPT > 120	8
Prior BMT or > 3 Rx	42
Donor type	
6/6 Related	37
5/6 Related	6
6/6 Unrelated	40
Preparative regimen	
FM180	65
FM140	12
CM180	6

CR1 = first complete remission, CP = chronic phase, BMT = bone marrow transplantation.

combined with melphalan 180 mg/m^2 (CM) as part of a randomized phase II trial. We closed this arm of the study early because of excessive toxicity; 5/6 patients died as a result of infection or multiorgan failure. GVHD prophylaxis was FK-506-based in 81 patients.

The median time to neutrophil recovery was 15 days (range 9–35 days) for recipients of cells from an unrelated donor and 13 days (range 11–25 days) for recipients of cells from a related donor. Platelet transfusion independence occurred in 30 recipients of cells from an unrelated donor and 28 recipients of cells from a related donor at a median of 21 and 16 days, respectively. The median percentage donor chimerism was 100 for both groups. Low levels of chimerism (< 50%) were seen in 2 patients who received cells from a related donor and 3 patients who received cells from an unrelated donor, including one patient with autologous reconstitution and one patient with secondary graft failure.

FM was significantly better tolerated than CM and was associated with a low incidence of grade III–IV Bearman toxicities (Table 4). CM toxicity was characterized by renal failure followed by multiorgan failure and occurred in 3/6 patients treated. GVHD was the major cause of death for recipients of cells from unrelated donors, while disease recurrence was the primary cause of treatment failure for recipients of cells from related donors. The incidence of acute and chronic GVHD is summarized in Table 5.

The 2-year survival for patients with AML/MDS was 36% and 40% for CML patients. Disease-free survival at 2 years was 34% for patients with AML/

Table 4. Number of patients with grade III–IV Bearman toxicities receiving melphalan/purine analog combinations

Regimen	Renal	Cardiac	Lung	Liver	NRM D30/100
FM (n = 77)	4/1	1/1	4/2	3/1	5/16
CM (n = 6)	2/3	0/0	0/1	0/1	3/2

Table 5. Incidence of acute and chronic GVHD in recipients of melphalan/purine analog conditioning regimens according to donor type

	All	Related	Unrelated
Acute GVHD II–IV	31/77	11/38	20/39
Acute GVHD III–IV	15/77	5/38	10/39
Chronic GVHD	24/45	12/25	12/20
GVHD deaths	17	5	12

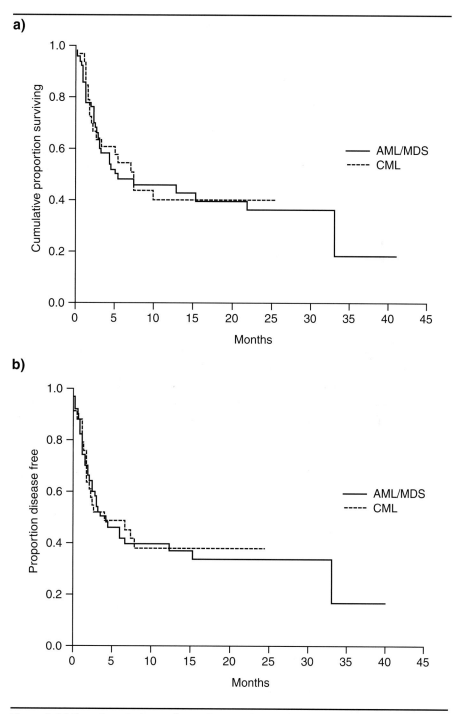

Figure 4. (a) Overall survival according to disease after melphalan/purine analog reduced intensity conditioning. (b) Disease-free survival according to disease after melphalan/purine analog reduced intensity conditioning.

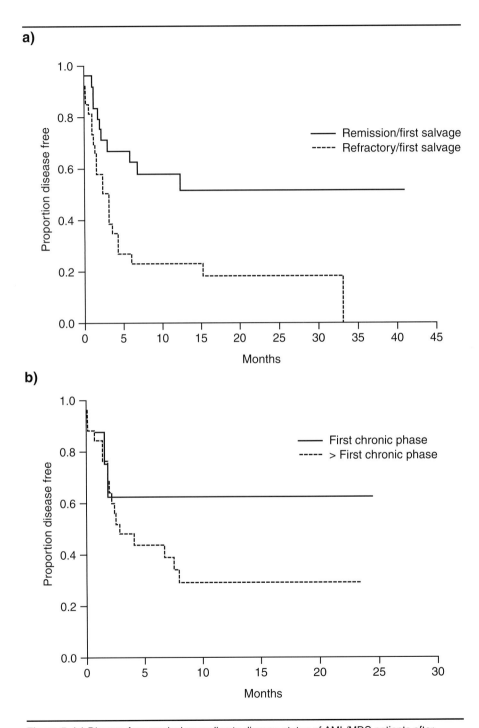

Figure 5. (a) Disease-free survival according to disease status of AML/MDS patients after melphalan/purine analog reduced intensity conditioning. (b) Disease-free survival according to disease status of CML patients after melphalan/purine analog reduced-intensity conditioning.

MDS and 38% for patients with CML (Figure 4). Disease status at transplant was the most important prognostic factor for disease-free survival, with patients with advanced disease doing significantly worse than patients treated earlier in the course of their disease (Figure 5).

In summary

This initial experience demonstrated that truly non-ablative therapies such as FLAG-ida are feasible in older and debilitated patients with myeloid leukemia. Results are encouraging if patients are treated early in the course of their disease. Further studies and formal comparisons with other standard approaches are warranted.

We have also demonstrated that reduced intensity conditioning with FM is well tolerated, provides sufficient immunosuppressive therapy to allow for engraftment of unrelated donor cells, and can produce similar long-term disease control in patients with myeloid leukemias considered poor candidates for conventional myeloablative therapies. GVHD and disease recurrence remain the most important obstacles to overcome.

References

1. Gale RP, Champlin RE. How does bone marrow transplantation cure leukemia? *Lancet* 1984; 2: 28–30.

2. Kolb HJ, Schattenberg A, Goldman JM, Hertenstein, B, Jacobsen N, Arcese W, Ljungman P, Ferrant A, Verdonck L, Niederwieser D. Graft-vs-leukemia effect of donor lymphocyte transfusions in marrow grafted patients. *Blood* 1995; 86: 2041–50.

3. Van Rhee F, Lin F, Cullis JO, Spencer A, Cross NC, Chase A, Garicochea B, Bungey J, Barrett J, Goldman JM. Relapse of chronic myeloid leukemia after allogeneic bone marrow transplant: The case for giving donor leukocyte transfusions before the onset of hematologic relapse. *Blood* 1994; 83: 3377–83.

4. Mackinnon S, Papadopoulos EB, Carabasi MH, Reich L, Collins NH, Boulad F, Castro-Malaspina H, Childs BH, Gillio AP, Kernan NA. Adoptive immunotherapy evaluating escalating doses of donor leukocytes for relapse of chronic myeloid leukemia after bone marrow transplantation: separation of graft-versus-leukemia responses from graft-versus-host disease. *Blood* 1995; 86: 1261–8.

5. Cullis JO, Jiang YZ, Schwarer AP, Hughes TP, Barrett AJ, Goldman JM. Donor leukocyte infusions for chronic myeloid leukemia in relapse after allogeneic bone marrow transplantation. *Blood* 1992; 79: 1379–81.

6. Drobyski WR, Keever CA, Roth MS, Koethe S, Hanson G, McFadden P, Gottschall JL, Ash RC, van Tuinen P, Horowitz MM. Salvage immunotherapy using donor leukocyte infusions as treatment for relapsed chronic myelogenous leukemia after allogeneic bone marrow transplantation: Efficacy and toxicity of a defined T-cell dose. *Blood* 1993; 82: 2310–8.

7. Rondón G, Giralt S, Huh Y, Khouri I, Andersson B, Andreeff M, Champlin R. Graft-versus-leukemia effect after allogeneic bone marrow transplantation for chronic lymphocytic leukemia. *Bone Marrow Transplant* 1996; 18: 669–72.

8. Tricot G, Vesole DH, Jagannath S, Hilton J, Munshi N, Barlogie B. Graft-versus-myeloma effect: Proof of principle. *Blood* 1996; 87: 1196–8.

9. Giralt S, Estey E, Albitar M, van Besien K, Rondon G, Anderlini P, O'Brien S, Khouri I, Gajewski J, Mehra R, Claxton D, Andersson B, Beran M, Przepiorka D, Koller C, Kornblau S, Korbling M, Keating M, Kantarjian H, Champlin R. Engraftment of allogeneic hematopoietic progenitor cells with purine analog-containing chemotherapy: Harnessing graft-versus-leukemia without myeloablative therapy. *Blood* 1997; 89: 4531–6.

10. Slavin S, Nagler A, Naparstek E, Kapelushnik Y, Aker M, Cividalli G, Varadi G, Kirschbaum M, Ackerstein A, Samuel S, Amar A, Brautbar C, Ben-Tal O, Eldor A, Or R. Nonmyeloablative stem cell transplantation and cell therapy as an alternative to conventional bone marrow transplantation with lethal cytoreduction for the treatment of malignant and non-malignant hematologic diseases. *Blood* 1998; 91: 756–63.

11. Khouri I, Keating MJ, Korbling M, Przepiorka D, Anderlini P, O'Brien S, Giralt S, Ippoliti C, von Wolff B, Gajewski J, Donato M, Claxton D, Ueno N, Andersson B, Gee A, Champlin R. Transplant lite: Induction of graft vs malignancy using fludarabine based nonablative chemotherapy and allogeneic progenitor-cell transplantation as treatment for lymphoid malignancies. *J Clin Oncol* 1998; 16: 2817–24.

12. Storb R. Nonmyeloablative preparative regimens: Experimental data and clinical practice. In *Educational Book of the 35th Annual Meeting of the American Society of Clinical Oncology.* Perry M (ed.). American Society of Clinical Oncology, Alexandria, VA, pp. 241–9, 1999.

13. Slavin S, Nagler A, Naperstek E, Varadi G, Ben-Yosef R, Panighari S, Samuel S, Ackerstein A, Or A. Well tolerated non-myeloablative fludarabine-based protocols for the treatment of malignant and non-malignant disorders with allogeneic bone marrow or blood stem cell transplantation. *Blood* 1999; 94 (Suppl. 1): 351a.

14. Giralt S, Khouri I, Braunschweig I, Ippolitti C, Claxton D, Donato M, Cohen A, Davis M, Andersson B, Anderlini P, Gajewski J, Kornblau S, Andreeff M, Przepiorka D, Ueno N, Molldrem J, Champlin J. Melphalan and purine analog containing preparative regimens. Less intensive conditioning for patients with hematologic malignancies undergoing allogeneic progenitor cell transplantation. *Blood* 1999; 94 (Suppl. 1): 564a.

15. Shimoni A, Anderlini P, Andersson B, Andreeff M, Braunschweig I, Claxton D, Cohen A, Donato M, Estey E, Gajewski J, Khouri I, Korbling M, Kornblau S, Molldrem J, Ueno N, Champlin R, Giralt S. Allogeneic transplantation for leukemia in patients older than 60 years: Age should not exclude treatment with non-myeloablative regimens. *Blood* 1999; 94 (Suppl. 1): 710a.

16. Childs R, Contentin N, Cleve E, Bahceci E, Hensel N, Boland C, Pomper G, Read EJ, Leitman S, Dunbar C, Young NS, Barrett AJ. Reduced toxicity and transplant related mortality (TRM) following non-myeloablative allogeneic peripheral blood stem cell transplantation for malignant disease. *Blood* 1999; 94 (Suppl. 1): 393a.

17. McSweeney P, Niederwieser D, Shizuru J, Molina A, Wagner J, Minor S, Radich J, Chauncey T, Hegenbart U, Maloney D, Nash R, Sandmaier B, Blume K, Storb R. Outpatient allografting with minimally myelosuppressive, immunosuppressive conditioning of low dose TBI and postgrafting cyclosporine (CSP) and mycophenolate mofetil (MMF). *Blood* 1999; 94 (Suppl. 1): 393a.

18. Kottaridis P, Chakravarty R, Milligan D, Chakrabarti S, Robinson S, Chopra R, Pettengell R, Marsh J, Mahendra P, Schey S, Morgan G, Williams C, Hale G, Waldmann H, Linch DC, Devereux S, Goldstone AH, Mackinnon S. A non-myeloablative regimen for allografting high risk patients: low toxicity, stable engraftment without GVHD, disease control and potential for GVL with adoptive immunotherapy. *Blood* 1999; 94 (Suppl. 1): 348a.

19. Khouri I, Lee M, Palmer L, Giralt S, McLaughlin P, Korbling M, Romaguera J, Donato M, Younes A, Ueno N, Gajewski J, Cabanillas F, Champlin R. Transplant-lite using fludarabine-cyclophosphamide (FC) and allogeneic stem cell transplant (alloSCT) for low grade lymphoma (LGL). *Blood* 1999; 94 (Suppl. 1): 348a.

20. Michallet M, Bilger K, Garban F, Attal M, Huyn A, Blaise D, Milpied N, Moreau P, Bordigoni P, Kuentz M, Sadoun A, Cahn JY, Socie G, Thomas X, Arnaud P, Lheritier V, Boiron JM. Allogeneic hematopoietic stem cell transplants after immune-ablative preparative regimen. A report of 92 cases. *Blood* 1999; 94 (Suppl. 1): 348a.

21. Niederwieser D, Wolff D, Hegenbart U, Mantovani L, Ponisch W, Deininger M, McSweeney P, Edelmann J, Kiefel V, Blume K, Storb R. Hematopoietic stem cell transplants (HSCT) from HLA matched and 1 allele mismatched unrelated donors using a nonmyeloablative regimen. *Blood* 1999; 94 (Suppl. 1): 561a.

22. Horwitz M, Barrett J, Childs R, Miller JA, Leitman SF, Read EJ, Carter CS, Linton GF, Malech HL. Non-myeloablative T-cell depleted allogeneic peripheral blood stem cell transplantation for patients with chronic granulomatous disease. *Blood* 1999; 94 (Suppl. 1): 710a.

23. Craddock C, Hughes T, Johnston R, Kreiter S, Bardy P, Apperley J, Goldman J, Derigs G. Engraftment of T-depleted allogeneic peripheral blood stem cells using a non-myeloablative conditioning regimen. *Blood* 1999; 94 (Suppl. 1): 394a.

24. Estey E, Plunkett W, Gandhi V, Rios MB, Kantarjian H, Keating MJ. Fludarabine and arabinosylcytosine therapy of refractory and relapsed acute myelogenous leukemia. *Leuk Lymphoma* 1993; 9: 343–50.

25. Kornblau S, Gandhi V, Andreeff M, Rios MB, Kantarjian H, Keating MJ. Clinical and laboratory studies of 2-chlorodeoxyadenosine + cytosine arabinoside for relapsed or refractory acute myelogenous leukemia in adults. *Leukemia* 1996; 10: 1563–9.

26. Sarosy G, Leyland-Jones B, Soochan P, Cheson BD. The systemic administration of intravenous melphalan. *J Clin Oncol* 1988; 6: 1768–82.

27. Singhal S. Powles R. Treleaven J, Horton C, Swansbury GJ, Mehta J. Melphalan alone prior to allogeneic bone marrow transplantation from HLA-identical sibling donors for hematologic malignancies: alloengraftment with potential preservation of fertility in women. *Bone Marrow Transplant* 1996; 18: 1049–55.

28. Li L, Keating MJ, Plunkett W, Yang LY. Fludarabine-mediated repair inhibition of cisplatin-induced DNA lesions in human chronic myelogenous leukemia-blast crisis K562 cells: Induction of synergistic cytotoxicity independent of reversal of apoptosis resistance. *Molec Pharmacol* 1997; 52: 798–806.

Non-myeloablative allogeneic stem cell transplantation for lymphoid malignancies using fludarabine-based regimens

C Hosing, IF Khouri

The term lymphoid malignancies describes a heterogeneous group of neoplasms that range from highly aggressive tumors to those with indolent natural histories. The lymphomas and chronic lymphocytic leukemia (CLL) have certain characteristics that make them attractive targets for treatment with allogeneic hematopoietic transplantation:

- they are highly sensitive to alkylating agents and radiation therapy, both of which are important components of preparative regimens for allogeneic transplantation
- they are associated with a steep dose–response curve.

Thus allogeneic transplants have been effective in producing durable remissions in patients with diffuse bone marrow involvement who have no other effective treatment options.

Considerable evidence indicates that high-dose chemotherapy alone is not effective in completely eradicating the disease in most patients with CLL or lymphoma. Instead an immune mediated graft-versus-lymphoma (GVL) effect is essential to prevent relapses.[1–4] Several studies have shown that allogeneic transplantation is associated with lower relapse rates in patients with CLL and lymphomas when compared to autologous transplantation using purged bone marrow.[5–9] In addition, it is possible to induce complete remissions in patients relapsing after allogeneic transplantation using immunosuppressive therapy[10,11] and by donor lymphocyte infusions (DLI).[12] Aggressive lymphomas appear to be less susceptible to GVL effects compared to CLL and indolent lymphomas.[9]

Compared to autologous transplantation, allogeneic stem cell or bone marrow transplantation for lymphomas is associated with higher complication rates and a higher transplant-related mortality (TRM) (usually in the region of 30–40%). This is primarily a result of the toxicity associated with the high dose conditioning regimens used, acute and chronic graft-versus-host disease (GVHD) and the associated risk of infections.[9,13] This risk increases with age and therefore allogeneic transplantation can be beneficial to only a subset of patients who are young and have a good performance status. Since the median age for diagnosis of CLL and lymphomas is 50–60 years, most patients will not be eligible for allogeneic transplantation using myeloablative regimens.

These observations led to the development of non-myeloablative conditioning regimens for allogeneic transplantation for the treatment of lymphoid malignancies (also called NST, mini-transplants or transplant-lite). The preparative regimen is not effective in eradicating the malignancy, but is immunosuppressive enough to allow engraftment of an allogeneic stem cell or bone marrow graft. The aim is to induce a state of mixed donor–recipient chimerism with minimal toxicity. *In vivo* expansion of immunocompetent cells after successful engraftment would be responsible for the GVL effect, which is an important component of allogeneic transplantation. We hypothesized that a less intensive preparative regimen would be associated with a lower TRM and could be used in patients who were not eligible for high-dose myeloablative regimens because of advanced age or comorbidities. In addition the risk of acute severe GVHD could also be lower in these patients because development of GVHD is in part related to the toxicity of the conditioning regimen and subsequent cytokine production.[14,15] The GVL effect may be augmented by the infusion of additional donor lymphocytes in patients who achieve successful engraftment.

The preparative regimen

The conventional-dose transplant regimen must be sufficiently immunosuppressive to allow engraftment of donor cells in the recipient's marrow and must also be able to provide tumor control early post-transplant to allow time for a possible GVL effect to be established. In addition the regimen must be minimally toxic, as indolent lymphomas are typically a disease of older and often debilitated patients. For these reasons fludarabine-based regimens were chosen. We conducted a phase I pilot trial using a combination of fludarabine and cyclophosphamide (FC)[16–18] (Figure 1) for indolent malignancies or a combination of cisplatin, fludarabine and cytarabine (PFA)[19,20] (Figure 2) for patients with aggressive histologies. These regimens are established frontline treatment

Pretransplant day	−5	−4	−3	−2	−1	0
	F	F	F			
	C	C	C			

F – fludarabine 25 mg/m²/day
C – cyclophosphamide 300–750 mg/m²/day
Day 0 – transplant

Figure 1. FC preparative regimen

Pretransplant day		−6	−5	−4	−3	−2	−1	0
		P	P	P	P			
				F	F			
				A	A			

P – cisplatin 25 mg/m²/day continuous infusion
F – fludarabine 30 mg/m²/day,
A – cytarabine 500–1000 mg/m²/day

Figure 2. PFA preparative regimen

regimens at M. D. Anderson Cancer Center (MDACC) for CLL and lympho-mas with an indolent or aggressive histology. They are moderately immunosuppressive and can be safely administered without hematopoietic pro-genitor cell rescue.

Patients were eligible for study if they were aged > 50 years or had other medi-cal comorbidities. All patients had failed to respond to or had recurred after primary therapy. Fifteen patients with a median age of 55 years (range 45–71 years) were studied. Eight patients had CLL which had relapsed after prior response to fludarabine (2 had undergone Richter's transformation) and seven patients had lymphoma (low-grade in 4, intermediate-grade in 3). Twelve pa-tients had active disease at the time of transplant, four had a performance status of 3 (according to Southwest Oncology Group criteria) and two patients had elevated liver function tests. All patients were heavily pretreated; the median number of prior chemotherapeutic regimens received was three (range 2–7). One patient had failed a prior autologous transplant.

Since the preparative regimens were known to be non-myeloablative, mixed chimerism was anticipated. Eleven out of 15 patients had evidence of engraftment as documented by the acquisition of donor type restriction frag-ment length polymorphisms (RFLP). The percentage of donor cells in the marrow ranged between 50 and 100% at 1 month post-transplant. One patient had 75% donor cells in the marrow at 6 weeks post-transplant but converted to 100% donor cells following DLI. The four patients who had graft failure re-ceived either the lower dose level of FC (3 patients) or PFA (1 patient). Hematopoietic recovery was prompt even in those patients with graft failure who recovered their autologous hematopoiesis. The regimen was well toler-ated and no patient had > grade II non-hematologic toxicity. All 11 patients who engrafted responded and eight achieved complete remission. We observed in this initial trial that complete responses can occur even in patients with mixed chimerism and that maximal responses are slow to develop and gradually oc-cur over a period of several months to a year.[21] These encouraging results have prompted phase II trials using non-myeloablative regimens for allogeneic transplantation in indolent and aggressive lymphomas.

NST in indolent lymphomas

Indolent lymphomas (diffuse small lymphocytic lymphoma, follicular small-cleaved cell lymphoma and follicular mixed small-cleaved cell and large cell lymphoma) account for 30–40% of all non-Hodgkin's lymphomas. The median survival of patients with indolent lymphomas is 8–10 years, however, these diseases are incurable with conventional chemotherapy.[22–25] High-dose chemotherapy with autologous bone marrow or peripheral blood stem cell transplantation in patients with relapsed or recurrent disease has produced disease-free survival (DFS) rates of 36–50% and overall survival (OS) rates of 65–70% at 4–8 years follow up.[26–28] For patients transplanted in first remission the DFS and OS rates are about 59–69% and 85%, respectively, at 4–5 years follow up.[29–31] The lack of prospective randomized studies, small number of patients in each study, different eligibility criteria and preparative regimens used makes it difficult to interpret the results. Therefore it is still unclear whether autologous transplantation provides a survival advantage when compared to standard dose chemotherapy in patients with indolent lymphomas. There is also concern regarding an increase in the risk of myelodysplasia and secondary malignancies in patients who have undergone autologous bone marrow transplantation, especially for diseases with a long natural history.[32,33]

Allogeneic transplantation has been studied in patients with indolent lymphomas. In a study of 113 patients published by the International Bone Marrow Transplant Registry in 1998, the probability of DFS at three years after allogeneic transplantation was 49% (95% CI 39–59%) and the recurrence rate was 16% (95% CI 9–27%). However, the 3-year TRM was 40% (95% CI 30–50%) and patients aged > 40 years were more likely to die from treatment-related complications (relative risk 1.85 versus 1.0, $p = 0.03$).[34]

Verdonck et al.[35] published a study comparing allogeneic and autologous transplantation in 28 patients with advanced low-grade lymphoma. The probability of disease progression among patients undergoing allogeneic transplantation was 0% versus 83% for autologous recipients at 41 months follow-up ($p = 0.002$). Progression-free survival was 68% versus 22% respectively at 2 years ($p = 0.049$). Similar results have been reported by others, who found an increased risk of relapse in patients undergoing autologous transplants even after B-cell purging when compared to those undergoing allogeneic transplants.[36] Since indolent lymphomas typically occur in older patients with other comorbidities most of them are not candidates for ablative high dose therapy. We therefore conducted a phase II study at MDACC[37] based on the results of our phase I trial[21] using conventional doses of fludarabine and cyclophosphamide as the conditioning regimen followed by peripheral blood stem cell transplantation in patients with recurrent indolent lymphomas. Patients aged < 70 years were included in the study if they had an HLA-identical sibling. Eleven patients with a median age of 51 years (range 36–67 years) were treated. They had received a median of 2 (range 1–6) prior treatment regimens and one patient had failed prior high-dose chemotherapy. At the time of transplant nine patients had sensitive disease and two had stable disease. One patient had evidence of active hepatitis C infection and one had renal dysfunction. The median duration of severe neutropenia was six days, which is about one week less than would be expected following high-dose chemotherapy. Eight patients never required platelet transfusions. Engraftment was achieved in all patients as documented by RFLP. The median percentage of donor cells in patient bone marrow was 80% (range 5–100%) at 1 month post-transplant. Toxicity was mild. No patient had a non-hematologic toxicity > grade II. Infection was limited to 3 episodes of fever of unknown origin. Only two patients developed acute GVHD limited to the skin (one patient had grade II GVHD and the other had grade III). The patient with grade III disease was treated with antithymocyte globulin and later developed chronic GVHD responsive to therapy. All patients achieved complete remissions and no relapses have been observed with a median follow up of 16 months (range 3–33 months). The observation that a durable remission could be obtained in patients who had a minimal amount of donor cells suggests that in indolent lymphoid malignancies, full chimerism is not needed to achieve optimal results.

NST in aggressive lymphomas

Aggressive lymphomas are highly responsive to combination chemotherapy and radiation therapy. About 30–50% of patients with newly diagnosed disease can achieve long term remissions. However the prognosis is generally poor in patients with recurrent or refractory disease.[38]

High-dose chemotherapy and autologous transplantation has been shown to improve the outcome in relapsed patients who have chemosensitive disease. In the PARMA trial, patients who underwent autologous stem cell transplantation had significantly better 5-year DFS (46% versus 12%, $p = 0.001$) and OS (53% versus 32%, $p = 0.038$).[39] Patients with refractory disease, multiple relapses or those with marrow involvement have a worse outcome; typically < 20% achieve durable remissions.

Several phase I and II studies have shown that allogeneic transplantation improves DFS rates in patients with aggressive lymphomas but this has been offset by a higher TRM. Use of peripheral blood stem cells instead of bone marrow is associated with accelerated hematopoietic recovery and may reduce the early TRM.[40,41]

In a phase II study conducted at MDACC, 15 patients with aggressive lymphomas (intermediate-grade in 8, mantle cell in 4 and CLL/Richter's in 3) were transplanted using the non-myeloablative regimen of PFA, as previously described.[42] The median age of these patients was 55 years (range 31–64 years) and all patients had received extensive prior chemotherapy (median number of prior chemotherapy regimens = 3, range = 1–6). All patients were ineligible for myeloablative regimens because of age or other comorbidities (prior autologous transplantation in 3, cardiac renal or pulmonary dysfunction in 3 and poor performance status in 2). Nine patients had stage III/IV disease at the time of transplant and 6 had disease that was refractory to (or untested with) salvage therapy. The regimen was well tolerated. The median duration of severe neutropenia was 3 days and the median requirement for platelet transfusions was 2 units. Fourteen of 15 patients engrafted with donor cells as documented by RFLP. More than 80% donor cells were present in the bone marrow of 6 patients at day 30 and 9 patients at day 100. One patient failed to engraft and another developed secondary graft failure. Eight patients achieved a complete remission (53%), 2 achieved partial remission (13%), 4 had stable disease or minor response (26%) and 1 patient had progressive disease (6%). At a median follow-up of 1 year, 9 patients (60%) are alive and 6 patients (40%) are in remission. Two of the five patients who relapsed went on to achieve a complete remission either after withdrawal of immunosuppressive therapy ($n = 1$) or treatment with rituximab ($n = 1$). Six patients have died (progressive disease in 2, GVHD post-DLI in 1, infection in 3). Early toxicity was mainly infectious (5 patients) and one grade 2 liver toxicity was observed. Two patients developed acute GVHD (grade 1–2) and 3 developed chronic GVHD.

This study demonstrates the feasibility of using non-myeloablative regimens and peripheral blood stem cell transplantation in patients with aggressive lymphomas. These preliminary results are encouraging given the patient population selected for the trial.

In summary

Pilot studies using non-myeloablative conditioning regimens for hematopoietic stem cell transplantation in patients with lymphoid malignancies are showing promising results, especially in patients with indolent lymphomas. GVHD has generally been mild and easily controlled using increasing immunosuppression. The minimal toxicity and mild cytopenias observed with the FC combination indicate the potential feasibility of this procedure in an outpatient setting.

References

1.	Gale RP, Champlin RE. How does bone marrow transplantation cure leukemia? *Lancet* 1984; 2: 28–9.

2.	Weiden PL, Sullivan KM, Flournoy N, Storb R, Thomas ED for the Seattle Marrow Transplant Team. Antileukemic effect of chronic graft-versus-host disease: contribution to improved survival after allogeneic marrow transplantation. *N Engl J Med* 1981; 304: 1529–33.

3.	Horowitz MM, Gale RP, Sondel PM, Goldman JM, Kersey J, Kolb HJ, Rimm AA, Ringden O, Rozman C, Speck B. Graft-versus-leukemia reactions after bone marrow transplantation. *Blood* 1990; 75: 555–62.

4.	Sullivan KM, Storb R, Buckner CD, Fefer A, Fisher L, Weiden PL, Witherspoon RP, Appelbaum FR, Banaji M, Hansen J. Graft-versus-host disease as adoptive immunotherapy in patients with advanced hematologic neoplasms. *N Engl J Med* 1989; 320: 828–34.

5.	Khouri IF, Keating MJ, Vriesendorp HM, Reading CL, Przepiorka D, Huh YO, Andersson BS, van Besien KW, Mehra RC, Giralt SA. Autologous and allogeneic bone marrow transplantation for chronic lymphocytic leukemia: Preliminary results. *J Clin Oncol* 1994; 12: 748–58.

6.	Rabinowe SN, Soiffer RJ, Gribben JG, Daley H, Freedman AS, Daley J, Pesek K, Neuberg D, Pinkus G, Leavitt PR. Autologous and allogeneic bone marrow transplantation for poor prognosis patients with B-cell chronic lymphocytic leukemia. *Blood* 1993; 82: 1366–76.

7.	Jones RJ, Ambinder RF, Piantadosi S, Santos GW. Evidence of a graft-versus-lymphoma effect associated with allogeneic bone marrow transplantation. *Blood* 1991; 77: 649–53.

8.	Mehta J, Powles R, Singhal S, Iveson T, Treleaven J, Catovsky D. Clinical and hematologic response of chronic lymphocytic and prolymphocytic leukemia persisting after allogeneic marrow transplantation with the onset of graft-versus-host disease: possible role of graft-versus-leukemia. *Bone Marrow Transplant* 1996; 17: 371–75.

9.	van Besien KW, Mehra RC, Giralt SA, Kantarjian HM, Pugh WC, Khouri IF, Moon Y, Williams P, Andersson BS, Przepiorka D, McCarthy PL, Gajewski JL, Deisseroth AB, Cabanillas FF, Champlin R. Allogeneic bone marrow transplantation for poor prognosis lymphoma: response, toxicity and survival depend on disease histology. *Am J Med* 1996; 100: 299–307.

10.	van Besien KW, de Lima M, Giralt SA, Moore DF Jr, Khouri IF, Rondon G, Mehra R, Andersson BS, Dyer C, Cleary K, Przepiorka D, Gajewski JL, Champlin RE. Management of lymphoma recurrence after allogeneic transplantation: The relevance of graft-versus-lymphoma effect. *Bone Marrow Transplant* 1997; 19: 977–82.

11.	Rondón G, Giralt S, Huh Y, Khouri I, Andersson B, Andreeff M, Champlin R. Graft-versus-leukemia effect after allogeneic bone marrow transplantation for chronic lymphocytic leukemia. *Bone Marrow Transplant* 1996; 18: 669–72.

12.	Kolb JH, Schattenberg A, Goldman JM, Hertenstein B, Jacobsen N, Arcese W, Ljungman P, Ferrant A, Verdonck L, Niederwieser D. Graft-versus-leukemia effect of donor lymphocyte transfusions in marrow grafted patients. *Blood* 1995; 86: 2041–50.

13.	Michallet M, Corront B, Hollard D, Gratwohl A, Milpied N, Dauriac C, Brunet S, Soler J, Jouet JP, Esperou Bourdeau H. Allogeneic bone marrow transplantation in chronic lymphocytic leukemia: 17 cases. Report from the EBMTG. *Bone Marrow Transpl* 1991; 7: 275–9.

14.	Antin JH, Ferrara JLM. Cytokine dysregulation and acute graft-versus-host disease. *Blood* 1992; 80: 2964–8.

15. Hill GR, Crawford JM, Cooke KR, Brinson YS, Pan L, Ferrara JL. Total body irradiation and acute graft-versus-host disease: The role of gastrointestinal damage and inflammatory cytokines. *Blood* 1997; 90: 3204–13.

16. Hochster HS, Oken MM, Winter JN, Gordon LI, Raphael BG, Bennett JM, Cassileth PA. Phase I study of fludarabine plus cyclophosphamide in patients with previously untreated low-grade lymphoma: Results and long term follow-up. A report from the Eastern Cooperative Oncology Group. *J Clin Oncol* 2000; 18: 987–94.

17. Keating MJ, O'Brien S, Kantarjian H, Plunkett W, Estey E, Koller C, Beran M, Freireich EJ. Long-term follow-up of patients with chronic lymphocytic leukemia treated with fludarabine as a single agent. *Blood* 1993; 81: 2878–84.

18. O'Brien S, Kantarjian H, Beran M, Freireich E, Kornblau S, Koller C, Lerner S, Kilbreath J, Keating MJ. Fludarabine (FAMP) and cyclophosphamide (CTX) therapy in chronic lymphocytic leukemia (CLL). *Blood* 1996; 88 (Suppl. 1): 481a.

19. Robertson LE, Pugh W, O'Brien S, Kantarjian H, Hirsch-Ginsberg C, Cork A, McLaughlin P, Cabanillas F, Keating MJ. Richter's syndrome: A report on 39 patients. *J Clin Oncol* 1993; 11: 1985–89.

20. Giles FJ, O'Brien SM, Keating MJ. Chronic lymphocytic leukemia in (Richter's) transformation. *Semin Oncol* 1998; 25: 117–25.

21. Khouri IF, Keating M, Körbling M, Przepiorka D, Anderlini P, O'Brien S, Giralt S, Ippoliti C, von Wolff B, Gajewski J, Donato M, Claxton D, Ueno N, Andersson B, Gee A, Champlin R. Transplant-lite: induction of graft-versus-malignancy using fludarabine based nonablative chemotherapy and allogeneic blood progenitor-cell transplantation as treatment for lymphoid malignancies. *J Clin Oncol* 1998; 16: 2817–24.

22. Horning SJ. Natural history of and therapy for the indolent non-Hodgkin's lymphomas. *Semin Oncol* 1993; 20 (Suppl. 5): 75–88.

23. Horning SJ. Treatment approaches to low grade lymphomas. *Blood* 1994; 83: 881–4.

24. Romaguera JE, McLaughlin P, North L, Dixon D, Silvermintz KB, Garnsey LA, Velasquez WS, Hagemeister FB, Cabanillas F. Multivariate analysis of prognostic factors in stage IV follicular low-grade lymphoma: A risk model. *J Clin Oncol* 1991; 9: 762–9.

25. Johnson PWM, Rohatiner AZS, Whelan JS, Price CG, Love S, Lim J, Matthews J, Norton AJ, Amess JA, Lister TA Patterns of survival in patients with recurrent follicular lymphoma: A 20 year study from a single center. *J Clin Oncol* 1995; 13: 140–7.

26. Bierman PJ, Vose JM, Anderson JR, Bishop MR, Kessinger A, Armitage JO. High dose therapy with autologous hematopoietic rescue for follicular low-grade non-Hodgkin's lymphoma. *J Clin Oncol* 1997; 15: 445–50.

27. Freedman A, Gribben J, Neuberg D, Mauch P, Soiffer R, Anderson R, Fisher D, Schlossman R, Kroon M, Ritz J, Nadler L. Long term prolongation of disease-free and overall survival following autologous bone marrow transplantation in patients with advanced relapsed follicular lymphoma. *Proc Am Soc Clin Oncol* 1997; 16: 89a.

28. Rohatiner AZS, Johnson PWM, Price CGA, Arnott SJ, Amess JA, Norton AJ, Dorey E, Adams K, Whelan JS, Matthews J. Myeloablative therapy with autologous bone marrow transplantation as consolidation therapy for recurrent follicular lymphoma. *J Clin Oncol* 1994; 12: 1177–84.

29. Freedman A, Gribben J, Neuberg D, Mauch P, Soiffer RJ, Anderson KC, Pandite L, Robertson MJ, Kroon M, Ritz J, Nadler LM. High dose therapy and autologous bone marrow transplantation in patients with follicular lymphoma during first remission. *Blood* 1996; 88: 2780–6.

30. Horning SJ, Chao NJ, Negrin RS, Hoppe RT, Long GD, Hu WW, Wong RM, Brown BW, Blume KG. High-dose therapy and autologous hematopoietic progenitor cell transplantation for recurrent or refractory Hodgkin's disease: analysis of the Stanford University results and prognostic indices. *Blood* 1997; 89: 801–13.

31. Martin D, Moos M, Voso M, Hohaus S, Ho AD, Haas R. High dose therapy with peripheral stem cell transplantation in patients with low-grade non-Hodgkin's lymphoma. *Blood* 1998; 92 (Suppl. 1): 460a.

32. Micallef M, Lillington DM, Apostolidis J, Amess JA, Neat M, Matthews J, Clark T, Foran JM, Salam A, Lister TA, Rohatiner AZ. Therapy-related myelodysplasia and secondary acute myelogenous leukemia after high-dose therapy with autologous hematopoietic progenitor-cell support for lymphoid malignancies. *J Clin Oncol* 2000; 18: 947–55.

33. Miller JS, Arthur DC, Litz CE, Neglia JP, Miller WJ, Weisdorf DJ. Myelodysplastic syndrome after autologous bone marrow transplantation: An additional late complication of curative cancer therapy. *Blood* 1994; 83: 3780–6.

34. van Besien K, Sobocinski KA, Rowlings PA, Murphy SC, Armitage JO, Bishop MR, Chaekal OK, Gale RP, Klein JP, Lazarus HM, McCarthy PL Jr, Raemaekers JM, Reiffers J, Phillips GL, Schattenberg AV, Verdonck LF, Vose JM, Horowitz MM. Allogeneic bone marrow transplantation for low-grade lymphoma. *Blood* 1998; 92: 1832–6.

35. Verdonck LF, Dekker AW, Lokhorst HM, Petersen EJ, Nieuwenhuis HK. Allogeneic versus autologous bone marrow transplantation for refractory and recurrent low-grade non-Hodgkin's lymphoma. *Blood* 1997; 90: 4201–5.

36. van Besien KW, Khouri IF, Giralt SA, McCarthy P, Mehra R, Andersson BS, Przepiorka D, Gajewski JL, Bellare N, Nath R. Allogeneic bone marrow transplantation for refractory and recurrent low-grade lymphoma: the case for aggressive management. *J Clin Oncol* 1995; 13: 1096–102.

37. Khouri I, Lee M-S, Palmer L, Giralt S, McLaughlin P, Korbling M, Romaguera J, Donato M, Younes A, Ueno N, Gajewski J, Cabanillas F, Champlin R. Transplant-lite using fludarabine-cyclophosphamide (FC) and allogeneic stem cell transplant (alloSCT) for low-grade lymphoma (LGL). *Blood* 1999; 94 (Suppl. 1): 348a.

38. Armitage JO. Drug therapy: treatment of non-Hodgkin's lymphoma. *N Engl J Med* 1992; 328: 1023–30.

39. Philip T, Guglielmi C, Hagenbeek A, Somers R, Van der Lelie H, Bron D, Sonneveld P, Gisselbrecht C, Cahn JY, Harousseau JL. Autologous bone marrow transplantation as compared with salvage chemotherapy in relapses of chemotherapy sensitive non-Hodgkin's lymphoma. *N Engl J Med* 1995; 333: 1540–5.

40. Ratanatharathorn V, Uberti J, Karanes C, Abella E, Lum LG, Momin F, Cummings G, Sensenbrenner LL. Prospective comparative trial of autologous versus allogeneic bone marrow transplantation in patients with non-Hodgkin's lymphoma. *Blood* 1994; 84: 1050–5.

41. Chopra R, Goldstone AH, Pearce R, Philip T, Petersen F, Appelbaum F, De Vol E, Ernst P. Autologous versus allogeneic bone marrow transplantation for non-Hodgkin's lymphoma: A case controlled analysis of the European Bone Marrow Transplant Registry data. *J Clin Oncol* 1992; 10: 1690–5.

42. Khouri I, Giralt S, Saliba R, Korbling M, Gajewski J, Younes A, Romaguera J, Anderlini P, Rodriguez MA, Donato ML, Ippoliti C, Keating M. 'Mini'-allogeneic stem cell transplantation for relapsed/refractory lymphomas with aggressive histologies. *Proc Am Soc Clin Oncol* 2000; 19: 47a.

Fludarabine with busulfan, cyclophosphamide or low-dose total body irradiation for non-myeloablative stem cell transplantation in matched siblings

S Slavin, A Nagler, M Aker, M Shapira, R Or

Introduction

Considering the limitations of a conventional bone marrow transplantation (BMT) procedure, which uses an aggressive conditioning regimen to eradicate the tumor or otherwise abnormal host cells, we have developed a new strategy that uses the BMT procedure as a platform for immunotherapy with allogeneic donor lymphocytes. This approach avoids or at least minimizes procedure-related toxicity and mortality as well as late complications, which ultimately may improve disease-free survival. This chapter reports the results from pioneering pilot clinical trials investigating the feasibility of non-myeloablative stem cell transplantation (NST).

Graft versus leukemia effects in clinical practice

Relapse following BMT can be reversed or prevented following infusion of donor lymphocytes (DLI) post-transplant.[1-5] Accordingly, DLI became an accepted modality for treatment of overt relapse as well as for the eradication of residual host cells escaping high-dose chemoradiotherapy following conventional myeloablative BMT. Interestingly, although graft-versus-leukemia (GVL) effects were originally documented in direct correlation with graft-versus-host disease (GVHD),[6,7] experimental and clinical observations suggest that significant GVL effects may also be accomplished in BMT recipients who have no clinically overt GVHD.[1-3,7-9] As was originally documented in mice,[10,11] resistance to GVHD improves as the time interval between BMT and DLI increases.[2,3,12,13] We therefore studied graded increments of DLI late post-BMT for treatment or for prevention of relapse post-BMT while partially controlling GVHD.[1-3,12]

Since maximally tolerated doses of chemoradiotherapy are unlikely to eliminate all tumor cells in patients with resistant or relapsing disease, and donor lymphocytes proved effective even in patients resistant to all available anti-cancer modalities,[1-3] it appeared that myeloablative chemotherapy might not be mandatory and could be replaced with adoptive allogeneic cell-mediated immunotherapy induced by alloreactive lymphocytes given at the time of transplantation, or supplemented with DLI following NST.

The development of NST

Myeloablative conditioning is not required for induction of stable chimerism.[15–17] Experiments using animal models showed that leukemia could be eradicated using immunotherapy mediated by alloreactive[8] or tumor-idiotype-reactive syngeneic lymphocytes.[18] This led to the development of NST in the early 1990s and a focus on cell mediated immunotherapy.[19,20] A number of protocols were developed, initially using escalating but non-myeloablative doses of cyclophosphamide and anti-T lymphocyte globulin (ATG) (Slavin *et al.*, manuscript in preparation). Subsequently, we introduced fludarabine into our NST protocols to intensify the pre-transplant immunosuppression and enable stem cell engraftment while avoiding the use of conventional myeloablative conditioning.[19–22] The first NST study consisted of increments of intravenous cyclophosphamide, starting at 50 mg/kg for 1–4 days following immunosuppression with rabbit ATG (Fresenius) used at 10 mg/kg for 4 days. NST was offered to patients with advanced malignancies (10 patients with hematologic malignancies and 7 with metastatic solid tumors) who were ineligible for conventional BMT. Durable engraftment was observed in patients who received at least two doses of cyclophosphamide. Three of 17 patients are alive and disease free > 5 years post-transplant (Slavin *et al.*, in preparation). Following this first NST study, we focused on the use of fludarabine-based regimens, with the goal of achieving acute immunosuppression for prevention of rejection of donor blood stem cells.

Fludarabine-based regimens

In Jerusalem, a number of fludarabine-based regimens have been studied:
- fludarabine 30 mg/m^2 x 6 days plus busulfan 4 mg/kg x 2 days (orally or more recently also intravenously), given in conjunction with ATG 5–10 mg/kg x 4 days (Figure 1) [19,22]
- fludarabine 30 mg/m^2 x 6 days with low dose cyclophosphamide (60 mg/kg x 2 days in patients with a normal immune system, or 5 mg/kg x 2 days in patients with Fanconi's anemia) and ATG (Figure 2)
- fludarabine 30 mg/m^2 x 6 days in combination with low dose total body irradiation (TBI) 200 cGy without ATG (Figure 3).[23,24]

Figure 1. Allogeneic NST for myeloid hematologic malignancies and genetic diseases from HLA matched siblings and matched unrelated donors

Days	−10	−9	−8	−7	−6	−5	−4	−3	−2	−1	0	+1
Fluladarabine (30 mg/m^2)	F	F	F	F	F	F						
Busulfan[1] (4 mg/kg)		B	B									
ATG (5–10 mg/kg)							A	A	A	A		
PBSCT or BMT											☯	☯
CSA/MTX[3]									C	C	C	

[1] Four doses of oral busulfan should be given to infants because of the unreliable intake and also faster rate of pharmacokinetics, alternatively intravenous busulfan could be used.
[2] Use as many stem cells as possible, preferably 2 collections of mobilized blood stem cells.
[3] CSA 3 mg/kg i.v. should be given starting on day −1 prior to transplant. Consider incorporating MTX 15, 10, 10 mg/m^2 on days +1, +3 and +6, respectively, to reduce the incidence of GVHD

Figure 2. Allogeneic NST for lymphoid hematologic malignancies, aplastic anemia and solid tumors from HLA matched siblings and matched unrelated donors

Days	−10	−9	−8	−7	−6	−5	−4	−3	−2	−1	0	+1
Fludarabine (30 mg/m^2)	F	F	F	F	F	F						
Cyclophosphamide (60 mg/kg)		C	C									
ATG (5–10 mg/kg)							A	A	A	A		
PBSCT or BMT[2]											☯	☯
CSA/MTX[3]										C	C	C

[1] In Fanconi's anemia use cyclophosphamide 5 mg/kg for 2 days
[2] Use as many stem cells as possible, preferably 2 collections of mobilized blood stem cells.
[3] CSA 3 mg/kg i.v. should be given starting on day −1 prior to transplant. Consider incorporating MTX 15, 10, 10 mg/m^2 on days +1, +3 and +6 to reduce the incidence of GVHD.

Following lymphoablation, granulocyte colony stimulating factor (G-CSF, 5 mg b.i.d. for 5 days) mobilized peripheral blood stem cells (PBSC) or bone marrow cells were infused. Low-dose cyclosporine (3 mg/kg/day) was administered from the day before transplantation and was discontinued 1–3 months post-BMT in the absence of GVHD in order not to block alloreactive donor lymphocytes and thus allow for the development of a graft-versus-malignancy (GVM) effect. More recently, we have added 3 doses of methotrexate on days

Figure 3. Allogeneic NST for high risk hematologic malignancies and metastatic solid tumors

Days	−7	−6	−5	−4	−3	−2	−1	0	+1
Fludarabine (30 mg/m²)	F	F	F	F	F	F			
TBI 200 cGy							TBI		
PBSCT								☊	☊
CSA/MTX²							C	C	C

¹ Use as many stem cells as possible, preferably 2 collections of mobilized blood stem cells.
² CSA 3 mg/kg i.v. should be given starting on day −1 prior to transplant. Consider incorporating MTX 15, 10, 10 mg/m² on days +1, +3 and +6 to reduce the incidence of GVHD.

+1, +3 and +6 post-grafting, in an attempt to better control the incidence and severity of GVHD. It was reasoned that the regimens should be applied in a disease-oriented way, therefore we used busulfan-based regimens for the treatment of myeloid malignancies and cyclophosphamide-based regimens for all lymphoid malignancies.

More than 150 patients were enrolled during the initial study period. Patients with an HLA-matched sibling and who had been followed for more than 6 months included:
- 74 patients with malignant myeloid disorders such as acute myeloid leukemia (AML), adult type and juvenile type chronic myeloid leukemia (CML), myelodysplastic syndromes (MDS), lymphoid disorders including acute lymphoblastic leukemia, non-Hodgkin's lymphoma, multiple myeloma, etc.
- 21 patients with a variety of non-malignant diseases such as beta thalassemia major, Gaucher's disease, Blackfan Diamond syndrome, severe aplastic anemia, Fanconi's anemia or infantile osteopetrosis (see Chapter 13).

All patients receiving an allograft from a matched sibling achieved durable 3-lineage engraftment (total white blood cells, nucleated cells, and platelets). Engraftment was rapid and most patients had 100% donor cells within the first 4–6 weeks post-NST. Some patients had detectable transient mixed chimerism; most patients converted to 100% donor type cells, either spontaneously or after discontinuation of cyclosporine A or, if indicated, following DLI.

The regimens were well tolerated and for many patients treatment could be given on an outpatient basis. Among the first patients analyzed, one third did not develop a nadir of aplasia, approximately 10% did not become granulocytopenic below 0.5 x 10⁹/L and approximately 10% required neither blood nor platelet transfusion throughout the post-transplant course. Following the non-myeloablative conditioning patients were maintained on oral intake, using a standard diet and only a few patients required parenteral nutrition. Mucositis was absent or very mild. The fludarabine + TBI regimen did not result in any hair loss and appeared to be the best tolerated regimen of those studied. GVHD was the single major problem in this series, with up to one third of the patients developing significant GVHD that was the primary cause of death in 14%. Nonetheless, the majority of the patients (56%) experienced no or only Grade I GVHD while on CSA. In some patients GVHD was activated when cyclosporine was discontinued or when DLI was attempted. Day 100 mortality was 4% for patients with hematologic malignancies and 2.6% when patients with non-malignant diseases were included in the analysis. The overall probability of relapse for the 74 patients with malignant myeloid disorders was 23%. To-date, with a follow-up of over 4 years, the probability of survival and disease-free survival is 58% and 42%, respectively. Out of 16 patients treated with DLI for recurrent disease, with or without prior chemotherapy, 11 responded. Other investigators, including Khouri et al.[21] who treated patients with low-grade lymphoid malignancies with fludarabine 30 mg/m^2 for 3 days and cyclophosphamide 300 mg/m^2 for 3 days, have confirmed these results. However, consistent engraftment was seen only when the dose of cyclophosphamide was increased to 750 mg/m^2 x 3 days,[25] which mirrored our earlier observations in patients treated with ATG and increments of cyclophosphamide. The combination of fludarabine 25 mg/m^2 x 5 days and cyclophosphamide 60 mg/kg x 2 days has been used successfully at the National Cancer Institute in Bethesda and by Childs et al. who used a fludarabine + cyclophosphamide-based protocol for the treatment of patients with metastatic renal cell cancer.[26]

The experience using NST in transplant centers other than the M. D. Anderson Cancer Center, Hadassah in Jerusalem and the Seattle Cooperative group is still limited. However, the feasibility of the original NST protocols has been studied elsewhere with promising results. Mayer et al. from Brno, the Czech Republic, used the NST protocol shown in Figure 1 with good results (personal communications). Bornhauser et al. from Dresden, Germany modified the regimen slightly; patients received fludarabine 30 mg/m^2 on days –6 to –2, busulfan 3.3. mg/kg i.v. on days –6 and –5. Patients with a matched sibling donor did not receive ATG while recipients of matched unrelated transplants did receive ATG (Merieux) 2.5 mg/kg for 4 days (personal communication). Many additional centers are currently applying one of the outlined NST regimens, with the majority using fludarabine-based regimens.

The data is not yet mature enough to draw any final conclusions, except to confirm that durable engraftment and rapid displacement of host with donor hematopoietic cells can be accomplished with well tolerated conditioning and low transplant-related mortality. Larger cohorts of patients and longer observation periods are required to fully assess the efficacy of NST in hematologic malignancies as well as in other potential indications for BMT. The optimal regimen needs to be defined and many questions remain to be answered, including, the intensity of pre-grafting versus post-grafting immunosuppression for controlling rejection and GVHD. The need for ATG or monoclonal anti-lymphocyte antibodies for the regulation of residual host T cells and/or alloreactive donor T cells to control GVHD should be investigated. Optimal methods for GVHD prevention, and delivery of DLI when required need to be defined.

In summary

NST allows engraftment of donor stem cells resulting in induction of transplantation tolerance to donor alloantigens. Engraftment of donor T cells present in the graft, or DLI administered following NST, can effectively eradicate otherwise incurable hematologic malignancies and life-threatening non-malignant diseases. NST is applicable to patients of all age groups and patients with a poor performance status. It appears from the existing cumulative experience summarized above that one of the major advantages of NST is that it produces a better immediate outcome, mostly due to no or shorter periods of pancytopenia, reduced incidence of side effects and improved resistance to bacterial infections, low incidence of mucositis, lower consumption of blood products and consequently lower procedure-related toxicity and mortality. For example, a young female patient treated with NST for AML in second remission gave birth to a female baby one year after the transplant suggesting that the reproductive system may be protected using non-myeloablative conditioning regimens. Furthermore, NST makes it possible to offer safer outpatient BMT procedures.

Based on the existing data and considering recent developments in basic and applied immunology, new horizons may be opened for safe clinical application of innovative immunotherapeutic procedures associated with adoptive allogeneic cell therapy. It is of paramount importance to understand and improve induction of transplantation tolerance to allogeneic stem cells by focusing on better immunoregulation and better control of host-versus-graft and graft-versus-host reactions. This may enable safer adoptive cell therapy of malignant and non-malignant diseases not curable with conventional modalities. Every effort should be made to include patients in clinical trials. This includes patients with minimal residual disease, preferably when still with good performance status, and patients who normally would not be eligible for conventional BMT protocols. Attention should be given to effective pre-transplant immunosuppression with minimal post-transplant immunosuppression to allow faster recovery of the immune system. Last but not least, since GVHD still represents the most serious hazard following NST and is the main cause of morbidity and mortality, better approaches for controlling GVHD are urgently needed, either through control of anti-host responses post-transplantation, by induction of graft-versus-host tolerance pre-grafting or by elimination of donor alloreactive T cells following induction of GVL or GVM effects.

We believe that non-myeloablative conditioning prior to stem cell transplantation, focusing on induction of transplantation tolerance as a platform for subsequent immunotherapy with immunocompetent donor lymphocytes has the potential to become the procedure of choice for the treatment of a large number of malignant and non-malignant disorders. The use of NST is accepted by many clinicians for elderly patients and for patients who may benefit from BMT not eligible for a conventional myeloablative procedure. However, it appears that NST will eventually open the field of stem cell transplantation to a larger number of patients in need, for a wider spectrum of clinical indications, with no upper or lower age limits. NST may therefore be considered for indications such as metastatic solid tumors, genetic diseases correctable by stem cell transplantation, life-threatening or drug resistant autoimmune diseases and immune deficiency disorders. It is therefore anticipated that NST may eventually provide a safer therapeutic option that may help accomplish the final goal of improved disease free survival and better quality of life for recipients of stem cell transplantation. Since AML as well as related myeloid malignancies such as CML and MDS are diseases that affect particularly elderly individuals not considered eligible for conventional BMT until recently, further studies towards clinical application of NST for this group of hematologic malignancies appears promising and should be further investigated prospectively on a larger scale, preferably by large cooperative study groups from transplant centers committed to experimental BMT and cell-mediated immunotherapy. In addition, a comparative trial comparing NST with conventional BMT with respect to long-term outcome may be warranted.

Acknowledgement

We would like to thank the following for their ongoing support: Baxter International Corporation; Max & Adi Moss Research Laboratory; Ryna & Melvin Cohen; The Szydlowsky Foundation; The Gabriella Rich Foundation. The work reported in this chapter was carried out at The Danny Cunniff Leukemia Research Laboratory.

References

1. Slavin S, Or R, Naparstek W, Ackerstein A, Weiss L. Cellular-mediated immunotherapy of leukemia in conjunction with autologous and allogeneic bone marrow transplantation in experimental animals and man. *Blood* 1988; 72 (Suppl. 1): 407a.

2. Slavin S, Naparstek E, Nagler A, Ackerstein A, Kapelushnik Y, Or R. Allogeneic cell therapy for relapsed leukemia following bone marrow transplantation with donor peripheral blood lymphocytes. *Exp Hematol* 1995; 23: 1553–62.

3. Slavin S, Naparstek E, Nagler A, Ackerstein A, Samuel S, Kapelushnik J, Brautbar C, Or R. Allogeneic cell therapy with donor peripheral blood cells and recombinant human interleukin-2 to treat leukemia relapse post allogeneic bone marrow transplantation. *Blood* 1996; 87: 2195–204.

4. Kolb HJ, Schattenberg A, Goldman JM, Hertenstein B, Jacobsen N, Arcese W, Ljungman P, Ferrant A, Verdonck L, Niederwieser D. Graft-versus-leukemia effect of donor lymphocyte transfusions in marrow grafted patients. European Group for Blood and Marrow Transplantation Working Party Chronic Leukemia. *Blood* 1995; 86: 2041–50.

5. Collins RH, Shpilber O, Drobyski WR, Porter DL, Giralt S, Champlin R, Goodman SA, Wolff SN, Hu W, Verfaillie C, List A, Dalton W, Ognoskie N, Chetrit A, Antin JH, Neumunaitis J. Donor leukocyte infusions in 140 patients with relapsed malignancy after allogeneic bone marrow transplantation. *J Clin Oncol* 1997; 15: 433–44.

6. Weiden PL, Fluornoy N, Sanders JE, Sullivan KM, Thomas ED. Antileukemic effect of graft-versus-host disease contributes to improved survival after allogeneic marrow transplantation. *Transplantation* 1981; 13: 248–51.

7. Horowitz MM, Gale RP, Sondel PM, Goldman JM, Kersey J, Kolb HJ, Rimm AA, Ringden O, Rozman C, Speck B. Graft-versus-leukemia reactions after bone marrow transplantation. *Blood* 1990; 75: 555–62.

8. Slavin S, Weiss L, Morecki S, Weigensberg M. Eradication of murine leukemia with histoincompatible marrow grafts in mice conditioned with total lymphoid irradiation (TLI). *Cancer Immunol Immunother* 1981; 11: 155–61.

9. Truitt RL, Shih CY, Lefever AV, Tempelis LD, Andreani M, Bortin MM. Characterization of alloimmunization-induced T lymphocytes reactivated against AKR leukemia *in vitro* and correlation with graft-vs-leukemia activity *in vivo*. *J Immunol* 1983; 131: 2050–8.

10. Slavin S, Fuks Z, Kaplan HS, Strober S. Transplantation of allogeneic bone marrow without graft vs host disease using total lymphoid irradiation. *J Exp Med* 1978; 147: 963–72.

11. Weiss L, Reich S, Slavin S. Use of recombinant human interleukin-2 in conjunction with bone marrow transplantation as a model for control of minimal residual disease in malignant hematological disorders. I. Treatment of murine leukemia in conjunction with allogeneic bone marrow transplantation and IL2-activated cell-mediated immunotherapy. *Cancer Invest* 1992; 10: 19–26.

12. Naparstek E, Or R, Nagler A, Cividalli G, Engelhard D, Aker M, Gimon Z, Manny N, Sacks T, Tochner Z, Weiss L, Samuel S, Brautbar C, Hale G, Waldmann H, Steinberg S M, Slavin S. T-cell-depleted allogeneic bone marrow transplantation for acute leukaemia using Campath-1 antibodies and post-transplant administration of donor's peripheral blood lymphocytes for prevention of relapse. *Br J Haematol* 1995; 89: 506–15.

13. Naparstek E, Nagler A, Or R, Slavin S. Allogeneic cell mediated immunotherapy using donor lymphocytes for prevention of relapse in patients treated with allogeneic BMT for hematological malignancies. In: *Clinical Transplants*, Cecka and Terasaki (eds.), Vol. 24, pp. 281–90, UCLA Press, 1996.

14. Johnson BD, Drobyski WR, Truitt RL. Delayed infusion of normal donor cells after MHC-matched bone marrow transplantation provides an antileukemia reaction without graft-versus-host disease. *Bone Marrow Transplant* 1993; 11: 329–36.

15. Slavin S, Strober S, Fuks Z, Kaplan HS. Long-term survival of skin allografts in mice treated with fractionated total lymphoid irradiation. *Science* 1976; 193: 1252–4.

16. Slavin S, Fuks Z, Kaplan HS, Strober S. Transplantation of allogeneic bone marrow without graft vs host disease using total lymphoid irradiation. *J Exp Med* 1978; 147: 963–72.

17. Slavin S. Total lymphoid irradiation (TLI). *Immunol Today* 1987; 8: 88–92.

18. Morecki A, Levi S. Puyesky Y, Slavin S. Induction of tumor immunity by intact irradiated leukemic B cells (BCL1) bearing a tumor-associated cell surface idiotype and the costimulatory B7 molecule. *Cancer Immunol Immunother* 1995; 41: 236–42.

19. Slavin S, Nagler A, Naparstek E, Ackerstein A, Kapelushnik Y, Varadi G, Kirschbaum M, Ben-Yosef R, Samuel S. Immunotherapy of leukemia in conjunction with non-myeloablative conditioning: engraftment of blood stem cells and eradication of host leukemia with nonmyeloablative conditioning based on fludarabine and anti-thymocyte globulin (ATG). *Blood* 1996; 88: 614a.

20. Giralt S, Estey E, Albitar M, van Besien K, Rondon G, Anderlini P, O'Brien S, Khouri I, Gajewski J, Mehra R, Claxton D, Andersson B, Beran M, Przepiorka D, Koller C, Kornblau S, Korbling M, Keating M, Kantarjian H, Champlin R. Engraftment of allogeneic hematopoietic progenitor cells with purine analog-containing chemotherapy: Harnessing graft-versus-leukemia without myeloablative therapy. *Blood* 1997; 89: 4531–6.

21. Khouri IF, Keating M, Korbling M, Przepiorka D, Anderlini P, O'Brien S, Giralt S, Ippoliti C, von Wolff B, Gajewski J, Donato M, Claxton D, Ueno N, Andersson B, Gee A, Champlin R. Transplant-lite: induction of graft-versus-malignancy using fludarabine-based nonablative chemotherapy and allogeneic blood progenitor-cell transplantation as treatment for lymphoid malignancies. *J Clin Oncol* 1998; 16: 2817–24.

22. Slavin S, Nagler A, Naparstek E, Kapelushnik Y, Aker M, Cividalli G, Varadi G, Kirschbaum M, Ackerstein A, Samuel S, Amar A, Brautbar C, Ben-Tal O, Eldor A, Or R. Nonmyeloablative stem cell transplantation and cell therapy as an alternative to conventional bone marrow transplantation with lethal cytoreduction for the treatment of malignant and nonmalignant hematologic diseases. *Blood* 1998; 91: 756–63.

23. Slavin S, Nagler A, Naparstek E, Varadi G, Ben-Yosef R, Panighari S, Samuel S, Ackerstein A, Or R. Well-tolerated non-myeloablative fludarabine-based protocols for the treatment of malignant and non-malignant disorders with allogeneic bone marrow blood stem cell transplantation. *Blood* 94 (Suppl. 1): 351a.

24. Slavin S, Nagler A, Naparstek E, Varadi G, Ben-Yosef R, Panighari S, Samuel S, Ackerstein A, Or R. A new non-myeloablative protocol using fludarabine and low-dose TBI in preparation for allogeneic blood stem cell transplantation for high risk patients with malignant and non-malignant disorders. *Blood* 94 (Suppl. 1): 388b.

25. Khouri IF, Lee MS, Romaguera J, Mirza N, Kantarjian H, Korbling M, Albitar M, Giralt S, Samuels B, Anderlini P, Rodriguez J, von Wolff, Gajewski J, Cabanillas F, Champlin R. Allogeneic hematopoietic transplantation for mantle-cell: molecular remissions and evidence of graft-versus-malignancy. *Ann Oncol* 1999; 11: 1293–9.

26. Childs R, Clave E, Bahceci E, Hensel N, Barrett J. Kinetics of engraftment in non-myeloablative allogeneic peripheral blood stem cell transplants: An analysis of hematopoietic-lineage chimerism. *Blood* 1998; 92: 520a.

Fludarabine and busulfan as non-myeloablative conditioning in high-risk second transplants and using matched unrelated donors

A Nagler, R Or, S Slavin

Introduction

Allogeneic stem cell transplantation (alloSCT) is the most effective modality to date for eradication of hematologic malignancies in patients at high risk of relapse or resistant to conventional doses of chemoradiotherapy.[1] However, high-dose myeloablative chemoradiotherapy is associated with a high incidence of transplant-related morbidity and mortality.[2–3] Alloreactive donor-derived T and natural killer (NK) cells have a major role in the anti-tumor effect induced by the graft, the so-called graft versus leukemia (GVL) effect.[4–7] The GVL effect may be safely achieved using allogeneic cell-mediated immunotherapy (alloCT) with donor derived peripheral blood lymphocytes administered in graded increments.[8,9] Moreover, tumor cells resistant to donor lymphocyte infusion (DLI) may still respond to interleukin-2 (IL-2) activated lymphocytes.[4] We have demonstrated that alloCT with IL-2 activated effector cells is a very effective modality for both treatment and prevention of relapse even in patients with resistant disease or at high risk of relapse.[10–12] Recently reported preliminary data also supports the existence of graft-versus-tumor (GVT) effect similar to the GVL effect. We have documented possible anti-tumor responses in 6 breast cancer patients with metastatic disease and 13 patients with advanced malignant lymphoma treated with donor lymphocytes obtained from an HLA-matched sibling. Donor lymphocytes were activated with rIL-2 *in vitro* and *in vivo*. One of the patients who when treated had no evidence of disease at the time of alloCT is still event- and disease-free more than 5 years after therapy.[13,14]

Based on this background, we have introduced the concept of non-myeloablative conditioning in which the bone marrow transplantation procedure is used as a platform for induction of host-versus-graft (HVG) tolerance rather than as a means of eradicating all tumor cells. Safe and stable transplantation tolerance can best be accomplished with the induction of mixed chimerism, which can be achieved using non-myeloablative conditioning. HVG tolerance allows consistent and durable engraftment of donor hematopoietic cells, so donor lymphocytes can be added if needed for induction of GVL and GVT effects to displace residual malignant or genetically abnormal host cells.

Using this approach for alloSCT of granulocyte-colony stimulating factor (G-CSF) mobilized peripheral blood stem cells (PBSC) from an HLA-matched sibling donor we were able to carry out a number of successful transplants. These transplants were well tolerated and were associated with low organ toxicity even in the older patients; the transplants resulted in fast and durable engraftment.[15]

Encouraged by these results, we decided to use a similar approach for unrelated bone marrow transplantation and high-risk second transplants. These types of transplants are associated with a high incidence of transplant-related complications, which are in part due to the intensified myeloablative conditioning that is generally used in this setting in order to achieve maximal immunosuppression and to ensure engraftment. We used our new non-myeloablative protocol as the preparative regimen for 16 consecutive patients with malignant disorders who received non-T cell-depleted marrow transplants and 9 patients who underwent second transplants for relapsing disease or secondary malignancy following autologous stem cell transplantation (autoSCT). Our results are encouraging, and suggest that non-myeloablative conditioning is sufficient to ensure engraftment with low transplant-related organ toxicity even in high-risk patients.

Matched unrelated non-myeloablative stem cell transplantation

Patient characteristics

Sixteen patients underwent unrelated bone marrow transplantation following non-myeloablative conditioning consisting of intravenous fludarabine 30 mg/m^2 x 6 days, busulfan 4 mg/kg x 2 days per os and intravenous anti-T-lymphocyte globulin (ATG) 20 mg/kg x 4 days. Seven patients had chronic myelogenous leukemia (CML), four had acute lymphoblastic leukemia (ALL), four had acute myelogenous leukemia (AML) and one had lymphoma. Two patients (one with AML, one with lymphoma) underwent non-myeloablative stem cell transplantation (NST) after relapsing post-autoSCT. Three of the patients were transplanted for secondary leukemia post-primitive neurosectodermal tumor (NPET), osteogenic sarcoma and malignant lymphoma. Thirteen of the patients were male and 3 female; the median age was 17 years (range 8–45 years). Two thirds of the patients had advanced disease.

Engraftment

All 16 patients engrafted, with no occurrence of early or late graft failure or graft rejection. Engraftment was durable and stable; 15 out of the 16 patients had 100% donor cells according to either amelogenine gene-PCR or VNTR-PCR techniques, which were carried out on the day of engraftment and once a month subsequently.[16,17] The median time post-BMT for the white blood cell count (WBC) to reach > 1.0 x 10^9/L was 15.5 days (range 8–23 days), for the absolute neutrophil count (ANC) to reach > 0.5 x 10^9/L was 17 days (range 11–23 days), and for platelets to reach > 25 x 10^9/L was 17.5 days (range 1–34 days). One patient did not have megakaryocytic engraftment.

Transplant-related organ toxicity

The incidence and severity of the transplant-related organ toxicity following NST was lower than that seen in our historical controls transplanted using a standard myeloablative protocol.[18,19] We observed only two cases of > grade II toxicity, according to the Bearman scale. One patient developed grade IV hemorrhagic cystitis with clots, which resulted in grade II renal toxicity and death 3 months post-BMT. Another patient developed grade IV undefined CNS toxicity and died 13 months post-BMT; a definitive diagnosis could not be made as the family refused brain biopsy. Grade II mucositis was documented in only three patients. All patients maintained oral intake throughout the procedure, with eight (50%) never requiring any parenteral calorific supplements. There were no cases of sepsis. There were no cases of pulmonary toxicity or multi-organ failure and no patient developed veno-occlusive disease (VOD) of the liver. Mild to moderate (grade I–II) transient disturbed liver or renal function tests were observed in nine and six patients, respectively. Two additional patients developed grade II CNS toxicity, including right focal seizures that responded to conservative therapy, and transient encephalopathy and behavioral changes (in a patient with grade IV graft-versus-host disease [GVHD]).

GVHD

Acute GVHD > grade II was observed in three patients: grade III in two patients and grade IV in one patient. The grade IV acute GVHD occurred in a 45-year-old patient with CML. This patient had received cyclosporin A (CSA) only as anti-GVHD prophylaxis in an attempt to consolidate a GVL effect as he was in accelerated phase (> 15% blasts in the bone marrow) at the time of transplant. On day +10 post-unrelated NST the patient developed hyperacute grade IV GVHD of the skin, gastrointestinal tract and liver, with hepatic encephalopathy. No improvement was seen following treatment with methylprednisolone, CSA, and subsequently with FK-506. The patient died 3 months post-NST. In the other two patients we observed transient grade III acute skin and liver GVHD that responded to standard steroid and CSA treatment. Four additional patients had transient grade II skin GVHD that responded to conventional anti-GVHD therapy. In all cases, acute GVHD developed while the patients were on CSA. No patient developed chronic GVHD during a median follow-up of 12 months (range 3–25 months).

Relapse

Three patients, two with ALL and one with AML, relapsed 9 months (range 5–17 months) post-transplantation. One of these patients was transplanted in relapse and one patient had secondary leukemia. These two patients received chemotherapy and donor lymphocyte infusion (DLI) and responded to treatment. The third patient with T-ALL and central nervous system (CNS) involvement has isolated CNS relapse 9 months post-transplantation and died. In all other patients with cytogenetic abnormalities we observed complete elimination of the malignant clones either by cytogenetic analysis or by disease specific reverse transcripts (RT)-PCR (e.g. bcr/abl in CML).

Cause of death

Three patients (18.75%) died of transplant-related complications. One patient who underwent matched unrelated NST as a second transplant for relapsed AML (as described above) died of severe grade IV hemorrhagic cystitis. An additional patient died of grade IV CNS toxicity 13 months post-unrelated NST. The third patient, a 45-year-old man in accelerated phase of CML, died of grade IV acute GVHD and hepatic encephalopathy. One patient (6.25%) died from relapse.

Survival and disease free survival

The actuarial survival and DFS rates at 12 months, according to the Kaplan-Meier method, were 75% (95% confidence interval [CI] 37–92%) and 70% (95% CI 36–88%), respectively. To date, after an observation period of 8 months (range 3–25 months), 12 of 16 patients (75%) treated with unrelated NST are alive, ten of them are disease free by all measurable criteria, including PCR and 11 patients are 100% donor chimeric.

Second allogeneic NST

Patient characteristics

Nine consecutive patients who were eligible for a second allogeneic BMT were included in this study. Five of the nine patients (three with lymphoma, one with AML, and one with ALL) underwent a second transplant for relapse following autologous ($n = 4$) or allogeneic BMT ($n = 1$). The other four patients underwent a second transplant because of secondary malignancy (three with AML and one with non-Hodgkin's lymphoma) after autologous BMT. The patients had received an autologous BMT for Hodgkin's disease ($n = 2$), lymphoma ($n = 1$) and breast cancer ($n = 1$), respectively. Seven patients were male and the median age was 37 years (13–63 years). The median time interval between the first and second transplant was 35 months (range 5–57 months). All the patients were transplanted from fully matched HLA-A, B, C, DR and DRB1 donors (seven sibling, two unrelated). All the patients were heavily treated and were transplanted in an advanced stage of their disease: four were in partial remission, four in full relapse and only one patient was in complete remission. The patients were conditioned for their second transplant with the fludarabine/busulfan/ATG non-myeloablative conditioning protocol described above. Patients transplanted from fully-matched sibling donors were given non-T cell-depleted G-CSF mobilized PBSC, while the two patients transplanted from fully matched unrelated donors received non-T cell-depleted bone marrow (BM) aspirates. PBSC were collected during one apheresis, after 5 days of administration of G-CSF 10 mg/kg/day in two divided doses.

Engraftment and chimerism

All the patients engrafted and no early or late graft failure was observed. The median time to reach a WBC of $> 1 \times 10^9$/L was 18 days (range 11–30 days), to reach an ANC of $> 0.5 \times 10^9$/L was 15 days (range 11–30 days), and for platelets to reach 25×10^9/L was 21 days (range 15–58 days). As described above, one patient did not have adequate platelet engraftment and developed severe protracted thrombocytopenia, severe hemorrhagic cystitis, and died. Engraftment was durable and stable and all 9 patients had 100% donor cells as confirmed either by amelogenine gene PCR or VNTR-PCR techniques.[16,17]

Transplant-related toxicity

The second NST procedure was relatively well tolerated when compared to the major toxicities seen following a conventional second transplant using standard myeloablative conditioning in historical controls[25] and reported in the literature.[25–31] Only three patients (33%) developed $\geq$ grade III treatment-related toxicities (Bearman scale).[20] One patient developed grade IV hemorrhaging cystitis as described above. Two patients (22%) developed grade III neurological toxicity that manifested itself as paraparesis and paraplegia. These two patients relapsed six and two months post-transplant, respectively, and died. Grade II mucositis was documented in four patients (44%). Five patients (55%) maintained oral intake throughout the post-transplant course, and two (22%) never required any parenteral calorific supplements. Mild to moderate (grade I–II) transient abnormal liver or renal function tests were observed in five and four patients, respectively; no patient developed severe VOD of the liver. Two patients (22%) who had lung involvement as part of their basic disease developed grade II pulmonary toxicity. There was no case of multi-organ failure.

GVHD

Acute GVHD > grade II was observed in only two patients (22%). In one patient, acute GVHD occurred 23 days post-transplant while they were receiving CSA. The patient experienced grade III skin and gastrointestinal tract involvement, grade II liver involvement and Grade I ocular involvement. Treatment with corticosteroids and CSA resulted in some improvement, however, the disease progressed to moderate extensive chronic GVHD involving the skin, mucosa and liver. The patient was treated with azathioprine and thalidomide and is currently (16 months post-transplant) under treatment with FK-506, showing good response and a Karnofsky score of 90%. The other patient developed acute GVHD 63 days post-transplant following rapid tapering of CSA in an attempt to maintain a GVL effect, since the patient was transplanted for AML in full relapse, secondary to breast cancer. The GVHD manifestations were grade III skin and gastrointestinal tract involvement, and Grade II liver and ocular involvement. The patient was treated with corticosteroids, CSA and anti-CD3 monoclonal antibody (OKT-3). The disease evolved into moderate extensive chronic GVHD of the skin, liver and mucosa. Treatment with azathioprine, thalidomide and phototherapy has resulted in some improvement, and, at the present time, 18 months post-transplant, the patient has a Karnofsky score of 80%. One additional patient had transient grade II acute GVHD and responded completely to corticosteroids and CSA therapy. One patient developed *de novo*, mild, limited skin and mucosal chronic GVHD 8 months post-transplant. The patient is being treated with low-dose corticosteroids and has a Karnofsky score of 90%.

Relapse

Three patients, who had aggressive disease and were exceptionally heavily treated, relapsed and died. The first patient had aggressive stage IV-A diffuse large-cell lymphoma, which was diagnosed in 1990. This patient underwent autologous BMT in 1992 and was in remission until relapse occurred in October 1995, with two large masses in the gastrointestinal tract and bladder, resulting in intestinal obstruction and massive hematuria. Surgery, irradiation and three courses of chemotherapy resulted in partial response. The patient then underwent a second transplant. However, 6 months later, the gastrointestinal tract mass recurred. The patient received involved field radiation, but died 3 months later. Two additional patients also suffered from aggressive malignant lymphoma. One of these patients had Hodgkin's disease stage III-B in resistant relapse with lung involvement. This patient underwent autologous BMT but relapsed and had a second transplant. Relapse again occurred 4 months after the second allogeneic BMT, and the patient was treated with alloCT consisting of DLI and IL-2, but died 8 months post-transplant. The second patient had lymphoblastic lymphoma with involvement of the CNS and lungs. The patient underwent a second allogeneic BMT for relapse 5 months after the first transplant, but relapsed 2 months later and died.

Causes of death

Three patients (33%) died as a result of relapse. Only one patient (11%) who underwent matched unrelated allogeneic BMT, died of organ toxicity (severe grade IV hemorrhagic cystitis)

Survival and disease-free survival

The actuarial survival and disease-free survival (Kaplan-Meier) at 23 months were both 48% (95% CI 16–75%). To date, with a median observation period of 12 months (range 7–23 months), five of the nine high-risk patients (55%) who underwent second transplant following non-myeloablative conditioning are alive and disease-free by all measurable hematologic and molecular criteria. Three have excellent quality of life and a Karnofsky score of 100%, while two have moderate chronic GVHD and a Karnofsky score of 90% and 80%, respectively.

In summary

Our studies suggest that durable and stable engraftment of donor hematopoietic cells may be achieved in heavily-treated patients with advanced malignant disease using a fludarabine-based non-myeloablative conditioning regimen followed by alloSCT. Since the chemotherapy in this novel conditioning regimen is of relatively low intensity (4 mg/kg busulfan x 2 doses), it is conceivable that the factor mainly responsible for engraftment is the immunosuppression induced by fludarabine in conjunction with ATG, and the relatively high number of CD34[+] cells in the peripheral blood infused at transplantation. Fludarabine is an effective immunosuppressive drug[21] that has been shown to synergize with ATG in promoting engraftment of megadose T-cell depleted CD34[+] purified haploidentical alloSCT across major HLA barriers.[22] Quesenberry et al.[23, 24] have already documented the feasibility of achieving bone marrow cell engraftment following syngeneic BMT with the establishment of mixed chimerism in non-myeloablated mice, when no transplantation barriers exist at all. Maximizing transient peri-transplant immunosuppression with the combination of fludarabine and ATG, and retaining donor alloreactive T-cells while avoiding high doses of conventional myeloablative chemotherapy and intensive post-transplant immunosuppression, may therefore be sufficient to ensure stable engraftment and elimination of residual hematopoietic cells of host origin while minimizing organ toxicity. In conclusion, the use of non-myeloablative conditioning makes it possible to achieve stable and durable engraftment, with complete or partial donor chimerism, while substantially reducing the incidence of transplant-related organ toxicity in high-risk second transplants and in transplants using matched unrelated donors.

References

1. Slavin S, Nagler A. New developments in bone marrow transplantation. *Curr Opin Oncol* 1991; 3: 254–71.

2. Thomas ED, Storb R, Clift RA, Fefer A, Johnson L, Neiman PE, Lerner KG, Glucksberg H, Buckner CD. Bone marrow transplantation. *N Engl J Med* 1975; 292: 832–43.

3. Thomas ED, Buckner CD, Banaji M, Clift RA, Fefer A, Flournoy N, Goodell BW, Hickman RO, Lerner KG, Neiman PE, Sale GE, Sanders JE, Singer J, Stevens M, Storb R, Weiden PL. One hundred patients with acute leukemia treated by chemotherapy, total body irradiation, and allogeneic marrow transplantation. *Blood* 1977; 49: 511–33.

4. Slavin S, Naparstek E, Nagler A, Ackerstein A, Samuel S, Kapelushnik J, Brautbar C, Or R. Allogeneic cell therapy with donor peripheral blood cells and recombinant human interleukin-2 to treat leukemia relapse post allogeneic bone marrow transplantation. *Blood* 1996; 87: 2195–204.

5. Collins RH, Shpilberg O, Drobyski WR, Porter DL, Giralt S, Champlin R, Goodman SA, Wolff SN, Hu W, Verfaillie C, List A, Dalton W, Ognoskie N, Chetrit A, Antin JH, Neumunaitis J. Donor leukocyte infusions in 140 patients with relapsed malignancy after allogeneic bone marrow transplantation. *J Clin Oncol* 1997; 15: 433–44.

6. Mackinnon S, Papadopoulos EB, Carabasi MH, Reich L, Collins NH, Boulad F, Castro-Malaspina H, Childs BH, Gillio AP, Kernan NA. Adoptive immunotherapy evaluating escalating doses of donor leukocytes for relapse of chronic myeloid leukemia after bone marrow transplantation: Separation of graft-versus-host leukemia responses from graft-versus-host disease. *Blood* 1995; 86: 1261–8.

7. Kolb HJ, Mittermuller J, Clemm CH, Holler E, Ledderose G, Brehm G, Heim M, Wilmanns W. Donor leukocyte transfusions for treatment of recurrent chronic myelogenous leukemia in marrow transplant patients. *Blood* 1990; 76: 2462–5.

8. Naparstek E, Or R, Nagler A, Cividalli G, Engelhard D, Aker M, Gimon Z, Manny N, Sacks T, Tochner Z. T-cell depleted allogeneic bone marrow transplantation for acute leukemia using Campath-1 antibodies and post transplant administration of donor's peripheral blood lymphocytes for prevention of relapse. *Br J Haematol* 1995; 89: 506–15.

9. Naparstek E, Nagler A, Or R, Slavin S. Allogeneic cell mediated immunotherapy using donor lymphocytes for prevention of relapse in patients treated with allogeneic BMT for hematological malignancies. *Clin Transpl* 1996; 281–90.

10. Slavin S, Naparstek E, Nagler A, Ackerstein A, Kapelushnik J, Or R. Allogeneic cell therapy for relapsed leukemia after bone marrow transplantation with donor peripheral blood lymphocytes. *Exp Hematol* 1995; 23: 1553–62.

11. Kapelushnik J, Nagler A, Or R, Naparstek E, Ackerstein A, Samuel S, Morecki S, Nabet C, Slavin S. Activated allogeneic cell therapy (allo-ACT) for relapsed chronic myelogenous leukemia (CML) refractory to buffy coat transfusions post-allogeneic bone marrow transplantation. *Bone Marrow Transpl* 1996; 18: 1153–56.

12. Toren A, Ackerstein A, Slavin S, Nagler A. Role of interleukin-2 in human hematological malignancies. *Med Oncol* 1995; 12: 177–96.

13. Or R, Ackerstein A, Nagler A, Kapelushnik J, Naparstek E, Samuel S, Amar A, Brautbar C, Slavin S. Allogeneic cell-mediated immunotherapy for breast cancer after autologous stem cell transplantation: A clinical pilot study. *Cytokines Cellular Molec Ther* 1998; 4: 1–6.

14. Or R, Nagler A, Ackerstein A, Kapelushnik J, Naparstek E, Samuel S, Amar A, Brautbar C, Slavin S. Allogeneic cell-mediated immunotherapy at the minimal residual disease stage following autologous stem transplantation for malignant lymphoma. *Immunotherapy* 1998; 21: 447–53.

15. Slavin S, Nagler A, Naparstek E, Kapelushnik J, Aker M, Cividalli G, Varadi G, Kirschbaum M, Ackerstein A, Samuel S, Amar A, Brautbar C, Ben-Tal O, Eldor A, Or R. Non-myeloablative stem cell transplantation and cell therapy as an alternative to conventional bone marrow transplantation with lethal cytoreduction for the treatment of malignant and non-malignant hematologic diseases. *Blood* 1998; 91: 756–63.

16. Pugatsch T, Oppenheim A, Slavin S. Improved single-step PCR assay for sex identification post-allogeneic sex-mismatched BMT. *Bone Marrow Transpl* 1996; 17: 273–5.

17. Nakamura Y, Leppert M, O'Connell P, Wolff R, Holm T, Culver M, Martin C, Fujimoto E, Hoff M, Kumliln E: Variable number of tandem repeat (VNTR) markers for human gene mapping. *Science* 1987; 235: 1616–22.

18. Nagler A, Brautbar C, Slavin S, Bishara A. Bone marrow transplantation using unrelated and family related donors: the impact of HLA-C disparity. *Bone Marrow Transpl* 1996; 18: 891–7.

19. Bishara A, Amar A, Brautbar C, Candiatti R, Lazarovitz V, Nagler A. The putative role of HLA-C recognition in graft versus host disease (GVHD) and graft rejection after unrelated bone marrow transplantation. *Exp Hematol* 1995; 23: 1667–75.

20. Bearman SI, Appelbaum Fr, Buckner CD, Petersen FB, Fisher LD, Clift RA, Thomas ED. Regimen-related toxicity in patients undergoing bone marrow transplantation. *J Clin Oncol* 1988; 6: 1562–8.

21. Keating MJ. Immunosuppression with purine analogues – The flip side of the gold coin. *Ann Oncol* 1993; 4: 347–8.

22. Aversa F, Tabilio A, Velardi A, Cunningham I, Terenzi A, Falzetti F, Ruggeri L, Barbabietola G, Aristei C, Latini P, Reisner Y, Martelli MF. Treatment of high-risk acute leukemia with T-cell-depleted stem cells from related donors with one fully mismatched HLA haplotype. *N Engl J Med* 1998; 339: 1186–93.

23. Nilsson SK, Dooner MS, Tiarks CY, Weier HU, Quesenberry PJ. Potential and distribution of transplanted hematopoietic stem cells in a non-ablated mouse model. *Blood* 1997; 89: 4013–20.

24. Rao SS, Peters SO, Crittenden RB, Stewart FM, Ramshaw HS, Quesenberry PJ. Stem cell transplantation in the normal non-myeloablated host: Relationship between cell dose, schedule and engraftment. *Exp Hematol* 1997, 25: 114–21.

25. Nagler A, Or R, Naparstek E, Varadi G, Slavin S. Secondary allogeneic peripheral blood stem cell transplantation (allo PBSCT) using a non-myeloablative conditioning regimen for malignant lymphoma (ML) patients who relapsed after autologous bone marrow transplantation (ABMT). *Blood* 1997; 90 (Suppl.): 550a.

26. Barrett AJ, Locatelli F, Treleaven JG, Gratwohl A, Zwaan FE. Second transplants for leukaemic relapse after bone marrow transplantation: high early mortality but favourable effect of chronic GVHD on continued remission. *Br J Haematol* 1991; 79: 567–74.

27. Wagner JE, Vogelsang GB, Zehnbauer BA, Griffin CA, Shah N, Santos GW. Relapse of leukemia after bone marrow transplantation: effect of second myeloablative therapy. *Bone Marrow Transpl* 1992; 9: 205–9.

28. Srivastava A, Gottlieb D, Bradstock KF. Diffuse alveolar haemorrhage associated with microangiopathy after allogeneic bone marrow transplantation. *Bone Marrow Transpl* 1995; 15: 863–7.

29. Boiron JM, Cony-Makhoul P, Mahon FX, Pigneux A, Puntous M, Reiffers J. Treatment of hematological malignancies relapsing after allogeneic bone marrow transplantation. *Blood Rev* 1994; 8: 234–40.

30. Kumar L. Management of relapse after allogeneic bone marrow transplantation. *J Clin Oncol* 1994; 12: 1710–7.

31. Arcese W, Goldman JM, D'Arcangelo E, Schattenberg A, Nardi A, Apperley JF, Frassoni F, Aversa F, Prentice HG, Ljungman P. Outcome for patients who relapse after allogeneic bone marrow transplantation for chronic myeloid leukemia. Chronic Leukemia Working Party. European Bone Marrow Transplantation Group. *Blood* 1993; 82: 3211–9.

Autografting followed by non-myeloablative stem cell transplantation for high-risk lymphomas

AM Carella

Among the hematologic neoplasia treated with allogeneic transplantation, the lymphomas appear to be particularly susceptible to a graft-versus-malignancy (GVM) effect.[1-4] Unfortunately the usefulness of allografting in the treatment of malignant lymphomas has been limited by the considerable conditioning-regimen-related toxicity. For example, the results in Hodgkin's disease (HD) have been disappointing;[5-8] mortality rates have ranged from 31% to 61%, with most series having more than 50% mortality.[8,9] In non-Hodgkin's lymphomas (NHL), allografting has yielded excellent relapse-free survival rates,[10-15] but the adverse effects of graft-versus-host disease (GVHD) have often negated this advantage so that overall survival is comparable to that seen with autologous transplants. For this reason, autografting is more frequently used than allografting in the treatment of lymphoma. The greater potential benefit of allografting could be exploited if conditioning mortality was decreased and tumor burden was minimized before conditioning. One way to achieve this is to use high-dose therapy with autografting to debulk the lymphoma, followed by an allograft using a non-myeloablative conditioning regimen (NST).

Between June 1997 and October 1999 20 patients with high-risk lymphoma who had HLA-sibling donors were enrolled on a NST protocol at the Department of Hematology of San Martino Hospital in Genoa. Details of each patient are presented in Table 1. Of twenty patients treated, 15 had been followed for more than 60 days. Ten patients (aged 19–36 years) had HD (6 Stage IVB, 2 IIIA, 2 IIA) and received their transplant a median of 22 months (range 7–120 months) after diagnosis. Status on entry was: 4 patients with primary refractory disease after 2–3 regimens, 1 patient in first relapse, 2 patients in second relapse, 2 in fourth relapse, and one patient in partial remission. Five patients (aged 24–60 years) had Stage IV NHL (Working Formulation A – 1; B – 1; E – 1; H – 2) and received their transplant a median of 25 months (range 6–121 months) from diagnosis. Two patients had chemorefractory disease, and there was one patient in either first, third, or fourth relapse, respectively. All 15 patients had a poor prognosis; the median number of prior chemotherapy regimens was 3 (including radiation in 10). Thirteen of the 15 patients had bulky mediastinal and/or retroperitoneal disease, and 2 patients had relapsed after autotransplants. All patients received cyclophosphamide (3 g/m^2) and granulocyte-colony stimulating factor (G-CSF) (5 mg/kg s.c. qd) to mobilize

Table 1. Patient characteristics

Patient number	Diagnosis	Age (years)/Sex	Stage	Sites	Time from diagnosis to ASCT (months)	Time from ASCT to NST (days)	Prior regimens
1	HD	22F	IVB	L	26	33	MOPP/ABVD, Dexa Beam
2	HD	36F	IIIA	Lymph node only	40	40	EBV/C-MOPP, CEP, RT
3	HD	26M	IVB	BM, MED	13	96	ABVD, EBV/C-MOPP, RT
4	HD	36M	IIA	MED	16	39	MOPP/AVBD, RT
5	HD	33M	IVB	L, MED	120	40	MOPP/ABVD, RT, CEP, VP-16 + EPI, Velbe, ABVD
6	HD	19F	IVB	BM, MED	16	40	ABVD, RT, MOPP
7	HD	32F	IIA	MED	18	40	ABVD, RT, MOPP
8	HD	34F	IVB	L, MED	54	114	MOPP/ABVD, RT, ABVD, CAV
9	HD	27M	IVB	H, MED	58	76	EBV/C-MOPP, RT, CEP
10	HD	36F	IIIA	MED	7	75	ABVD, MOPP/ABVD, MOPP
11	NHL	43M	IVA/WF:A	BM/RPT	25	62	fludarabine + idarubicin, CNOP
12	NHL	24F	IVA/WF:H	L, H, K, MED	6	62	CHOP, VP-16+EPI, MACOP-B
13	NHL	60M	IVB/WF:E	L, BM, MED, RPT	121	61	fludarabine + idarubicin,CNOP, RT, B-CEPP, DHAP, fludarabine + idarubicin
14	NHL	40M	IVA/WF:B	L, MED	15	210	CVP
15	NHL	48F	IVB/WF:H	L, H, RPT	28	40	MACOP-B, DHAP, RT, ASCT

MED: Mediastinal bulk; RPT: Retroperitoneal bulk; L: Lung; BM: Bone marrow; H: Liver; K: Kidney; ASCT: Autologous stem cell transplantation; RT: Radiotherapy hematopoietic stem cells (HSC) and CD34[+] cells were obtained by leukapheresis and cryopreserved. The preparative regimen for autografting was the BEAM protocol (carmustine 300 mg/m^2 day 1, etoposide 200 mg/m^2 days 2–5, arabinosylcytosine 200 mg/m^2 b.i.d. days 2–5 and melphalan 140 mg/m^2 on day 6). Two or three days after chemotherapy, autologous HSC were reinfused into the patients. Following a brief recovery period, patients were discharged and their response monitored. When clinically stable, patients were readmitted for allogeneic transplant a median of 61 days (range 33–210 days) after autografting. The preparative regimen consisted of fludarabine 30 mg/m^2 followed by cyclophosphamide 300 mg/m^2 (FC) on days –4, –3, –2 prior to infusion of donor cells. Methotrexate (8 mg/m^2 on day +1, +3, +5) and cyclosporine (CSA) were used to prevent graft rejection and as GVHD prophylaxis. CSA was given from day –1, initially at an intravenous dose of 1 mg/kg daily (which was later changed to 5 mg/kg orally), and continued through to day +90. Donors received 10 mg/kg G-CSF daily for 3–4 days. Mobilized HSC were collected by leukapheresis on day +5 and again on day +6, if necessary, to achieve a dose of $\geq$ 2 x 10^6 CD34[+] cells/kg of recipient weight. Donor collections were prepared for fresh infusion and were not T cell depleted, but in cases of major or minor ABO incompatibility between donor and recipient were subjected to standard procedures for erythrocyte or plasma removal, respectively. On day 0 (and on day +1 if required) unmanipulated HSC were transfused to the recipients. Patients showing 100% donor complete chimerism by mini-satellite analysis on day +45 continued CSA until day +100; thereafter CSA was tapered by 25–30% every 7–10 days and discontinued if no sign of GVHD developed. CSA was tapered off over 7–10 days in patients with mixed chimerism on day +45, and chimerism analysis was repeated weekly. Patients not converting to 100% donor chimerism after CSA withdrawal received monthly escalating doses of DLI (1 x 10^6/kg, 1 x 10^7/kg, 5 x 10^7/kg) with weekly evaluation of chimerism until 100% donor chimerism, GVHD, disease regression, or graft rejection occurred. Patients with symptomatic acute GVHD were treated with CSA and methylprednisolone. In all patients, serial samples of bone marrow were analyzed for the degree of donor–recipient chimerism using a polymerase chain reaction (PCR) assay of informative minisatellite regions.

Results

The outcome of 15 patients undergoing autografting followed by NST are listed in Table 2. All patients tolerated the BEAM protocol well and no serious complication other than mucositis was observed. All 5 patients with NHL obtained a partial remission of lymphoma on computerized tomography (CT) scan.

Table 2. Results in the different phases of treatment

Patient number	Status pre-ASCT	Status post-ASCT	Status post-NST	BM chimerism 100% donor (days)	Outcome (days)
1	PRD	PR	PD	210*	Died PD/cGvHD (Liver)(460)
2	Rel-2	PR	CR3	90*	Alive/Rel-4 grade II aGVHD (> 700)
3	PRD	PR	PD	–	Died PD (66)
4	Rel-2	PR	CR3	–	Died in CR3, grade III aGVHD (brain Aspergillus)(120)
5	Rel-4	CR5	PR	420*	Alive PR grade III aGVHD (> 600)
6	PR	CR1*	CR2	410*	Alive CR2 grade I aGVHD (> 430)
7	Rel-1	CR2	CR2	210*	Alive CR2 (>300)
8	PRD	PR	CR1	115	Alive CR1 (>335)
9	Rel-4	PR	CR5	307	Alive CR5, grade III aGVHD (>340)
10	PRD	PR	CR1	150	Alive CR1, grade II aGVHD (>210)
11	PRD	PR	CR1	150	Alive Rel-2, grade I aGVHD (>630)
12	PRD	PR	PD	90	Died PD grade II aGVHD (172)
13	Rel-4	PR	CR5	150*	Died in CR5/extensive cGVHD (260)
14	Rel-1	PR	CR2	90*	Alive CR2 (>240)
15	Rel-3	PR	CR4	115	Alive CR4 grade II aGVHD (>270)

PR: Partial remission; CR: Complete remission; Rel: Relapse; PD: Progressive disease; ASCT: Autologous stem cell transplantation; PRD: Primary refractory disease
*After DLI

Among the 10 HD patients, three obtained a complete remission with disappearance of their disease in bone marrow, mediastinal and/or lung. Six patients obtained partial remission (40–60% reduction of mediastinal bulky, lung and liver localizations) and one patient had no response.

The allografting admission began < 62 days post-autografting in 10 patients (6 HD, 4 NHL). This process was delayed in five patients (4 HD, 1 NHL) until 75–210 days post-autograft due to the presence of persistent thrombocytopenia. Apart from transient nausea in 2 patients, the FC regimen was well-tolerated with no mucositis or hemorrhagic cystitis. All patients were managed in conventional rooms. The patients were discharged after a median of 18 days (range 3–25 days) and the last five patients received the preparative regimen as outpatients. Three patients were positive for cytomegalovirus antigenemia and were treated successfully with ganciclovir.

Ten patients were in complete remission after allografting. Two (CR1 and CR5) of the three patients in remission after autografting relapsed before mini-allografting. One of them achieved a new CR (CR2) after three courses of MOPP and maintained this remission 430 days after allografting. The second patient achieved partial remission after allografting and is alive and in partial remission 600 days post-transplant. The last patient maintained the CR that was achieved after autografting (330 days). Eight patients who were in partial remission after autografting achieved a complete remission after allografting (CR1 = 3, CR2 = 1, CR3 = 2, CR4 = 1, CR5 = 1). In total, 4/5 patients with NHL and 6/10 with HD achieved a complete remission with this protocol.

Chimerism analysis

All patients had evidence of donor cell engraftment, as documented by short tandem repeats in the bone marrow on day 30. The percentage of donor cells increased progressively on subsequent marrows and six patients achieved complete donor chimerism 90–210 days (median 133 days) post-NST. Subsequently, two of these patients received DLI in order to control the progression of disease; one patient returned to mixed chimerism. Seven of the remaining patients with mixed chimerism received a DLI beginning on day 60 (one patient), day 90 (4 patients), day 150 (one patient) or day 300 (one patient) post-transplant. DLI resulted in full chimerism in five patients. Prior to receiving DLI, grade I–II acute GVHD of the skin and gastrointestinal tract occurred in 2 patients; another patient developed grade III GVHD of the gastrointestinal tract and grade II acute GVHD of the skin. The course in this patient was complicated by bacterial aspergillus pneumonia, which resolved, but thereafter the HD relapsed and the patient died as a result of extensive chronic GVHD and HD at 460 days post-transplant. After DLI, 6/7 patients developed acute GVHD (skin/gastrointestinal tract grade ≤ II in 4 patients; grade III in 2 patients).

Eleven patients survive 210–780 days (median 330 days) post-transplant. Five patients died, two of progressive disease, two of progressive disease and extensive chronic GVHD and one patient of brain hemorrhage following aspergillus infection in whom an autopsy revealed continued complete remission.

In summary

The 15 patients in this study were unlikely to be cured with autografting alone. After autografting, three patients achieved complete remission but two of them relapsed shortly before the NST. All other patients were in partial remission at the time of the allografting procedure. Allografting with non-myeloablative conditioning produced remissions in eight of these patients, three of whom achieved remission for the first time. These results emphasize the central role of the GVL effect in mediating this dramatic lymphoma regression. Complete chimerism was documented in eleven patients after day +90, five without DLI and six after a series of DLI. The experience in these patients with high-risk lymphoma demonstrates that this combined procedure is feasible.

References

1. Rondòn G, Giralt S, Huh Y, Khouri I, Andersson B, Andreeff M, Champlin R. Graft-versus-leukemia effect after allogeneic bone marrow transplantation for chronic lymphocytic leukemia. *Bone Marrow Transpl* 1996; 18: 669–72.

2. van Besien K, Sobocinski KA, Rowlings PA, Murphy SC, Armitage JO, Bishop MR, Chaekal OK, Gale RP, Klein JP, Lazarus HM, McCarthy PL Jr, Raemaekers JM, Reiffers J, Phillips GL, Schattenberg AV, Verdonck LF, Vose JM, Horowitz MM. Allogeneic bone marrow transplantation for low-grade lymphoma. *Blood* 1998; 92: 1832–6.

3. Khouri IF, Przepiorka D, Van Besien K, O'Brien S, Palmer JL, Lerner S, Mehra RC, Vriesendorp HM, Andersson BS, Giralt S, Korbling M, Keating MJ, Champlin RE. Allogeneic blood or marrow transplantation for chronic lymphocytic leukaemia: Timing of transplantation and potential effect of fludarabine on acute graft-versus-host disease. *Br J Haematol* 1997; 97: 466–73.

4. Tricot G, Vesole DH, Jagannath S, Hilton J, Munshi N, Barlogie B. Graft-versus-myeloma effect: Proof of principle. *Blood* 1996; 87: 1196–8.

5. Milpied N, Fielding AK, Pearce RM, Ernst P, Goldstone AH. Allogeneic bone marrow transplant is not better than autologous transplant for patients with relapsed Hodgkin's disease. *J Clin Oncol* 1996; 14: 1291–6.

6. Anderson JE, Litzow MR, Appelbaum FR, Schoch G, Fisher LD, Buckner CD, Petersen FB, Crawford SW, Press OW, Sanders JE. Allogeneic syngeneic and autologous marrow transplantation for Hodgkin's disease: the 21-year Seattle experience. *J Clin Oncol* 1993; 11: 2342–50.

7. Jones RJ, Piantadosi S, Mann RB, Ambinder RF, Seifter EJ, Vriesendorp HM, Abeloff MD, Burns WH, May WS, Rowley SD. High-dose cytotoxic therapy and bone marrow transplantation for relapsed Hodgkin's disease. *J Clin Oncol* 1990; 8: 527–37.

8. Armitage JO, Goldstone AH, Carella AM, *et al.* Role of bone marrow transplantation in Hodgkin's Disease. In: *Hodgkin's Disease*, Mauch PM, Armitage JO, Diehl V, Hoppe RT and Weiss LM (eds), Lippincott Williams and Wilkins, Philadelphia 1999, pp. 521–30.

9. Gajewski JL, Phillips GL, Sobocinski KA, Armitage JO, Gale RP, Champlin RE, Herzig RH, Hurd DD, Jagannath S, Klein JP, Lazarus HM, McCarthy PL Jr, Pavlovsky S, Peterson FB, Rowlings PA, Russell JA, Silver SM, Vose JM, Wiernik PH, Bortin MM, Horowitz MM. Bone marrow transplants from HLA-identical siblings in advanced Hodgkin's disease. *J Clin Oncol* 1996; 14: 572–8.

10. Jones RJ, Ambinder RF, Piantadosi S, Santos GW. Evidence of a graft-versus-lymphoma effect associated with allogeneic bone marrow transplantation. *Blood* 1991; 3: 649–53.

11. Chopra R, Goldstone AH, Pearce R, Philip T, Petersen F, Appelbaum F, De Vol E, Ernst P. Autologous versus allogeneic bone marrow transplantation for non-Hodgkin's lymphoma: a case-controlled analysis of the European Bone Marrow Transplant Group registry data. *J Clin Oncol* 1992; 11: 1690–5.

12. van Besien KW, Mehra RC, Giralt SA, Kantarjian HM, Pugh WC, Khouri IF, Moon Y, Williams P, Andersson BS, Przepiorka D, McCarthy PL, Gajewski JL, Deisseroth AB, Cabanillas FF, Champlin R. Allogeneic bone marrow transplantation for poor-prognosis lymphoma: response, toxicity and survival depend on disease histology. *Am J Med* 1996; 100: 299–307.

13. Ratanatharathorn V, Uberti J, Karanes C, Abella E, Lum LG, Momin F, Cummings G, Sensenbrenner LL. Prospective comparative trial of autologous versus allogeneic bone marrow transplantation in patients with non-Hodgkin's lymphoma. *Blood* 1994; 84: 1050–5.

14.   Appelbaum FR. Treatment of aggressive non-Hodgkin's lymphoma with marrow transplantation. *Marrow Transplant Rev* 1993; 3: 1.

15.   Verdonck LF, Dekker AW, Lokhorst HM, Petersen EJ, Nieuwenhuis HK. Allogeneic versus autologous bone marrow transplantation for refractory and recurrent low grade non-Hodgkin's lymphoma. *Blood* 1997; 90: 4201–5.

Graft-versus-tumor effects following non-myeloablative stem cell transplantation

R Childs, J Barrett

Introduction

The observation that potent and durable anti-leukemic effects occur against a variety of hematologic malignancies following allogeneic stem cell transplantation raises the question of whether a similar beneficial allo-response might be inducible against non-hematologic malignancies.[1–7] The high risk of treatment-related mortality associated with conventional 'high-dose' myeloablative transplants has largely precluded any systematic investigation of a graft-versus-solid tumor (GVT) effect. Non-myeloablative stem cell transplantation (NST) has quickly proven to be a safer alternative to conventional allogeneic blood or marrow transplantation (BMT) for the safe delivery of an allogeneic immune system for the investigation of GVT effects in patients with otherwise incurable metastatic solid tumors.[8–13]

In theory, all carcinomas arising from epithelial tissues, which are involved in either acute or chronic graft-versus-host disease (GVHD) (i.e. keratinocytes, fibroblasts, exocrine glands, hepatobiliary tree, gastrointestinal tract) should be susceptible to a GVT effect. From our understanding of graft-versus-leukemia, the tumor cell characteristics necessary to generate a successful GVT response would include susceptibility to lysis by allogeneic cytotoxic T cells (CTL) or natural killer (NK)/lymphokine-activated killer (LAK) cells, slow proliferation (matching the relatively slow pace of the T-cell response), and presence of major histocompatability complex (MHC) molecules on the cell surface. Many tumors possess some or all of these characteristics. However, it should be noted that solid tumors might also be well adapted to escape immune-mediated killing. Locus or allele-specific downregulation of MHC molecules is a common mechanism whereby tumor cells escape T cell attack.[14, 15] Increased concentrations of membrane-bound Fas-ligand[16] as well as tumor release of soluble inhibitory factors such as IL-10, transforming growth factor beta (TGF-β),[17] or soluble inhibitors of nuclear factor kappaB (NFκB) may all inhibit an allogeneic immune mediated cytotoxic effect.

Transplant approach

In designing allogeneic transplantation protocols for patients with tumors not susceptible to dose intensification, it seems logical to minimize the risk of regimen-related toxicity by reducing the intensity of the conditioning regimen. There is a theoretical risk that immunosuppression given to establish engraftment of the donor cells may actually accelerate disease progression in tumors being held in check by the recipient's immune system. For this reason, a prudent approach to allografting patients with tumors would be to use a T cell replete allograft in order to establish complete and rapid donor immune reconstitution. Furthermore, to enhance the chances of establishing a GVT effect, GVHD prophylactic drugs (i.e. FK-506 and cyclosporine [CSA]) should be withdrawn early, and if required, donor lymphocytes given (Figure 1). Other modalities that might enhance GVT post-transplant include the use of interferons to up-regulate MHC and co-stimulatory molecules on the tumor, IL-2 to enhance T-cell and NK cell responses, and granulocyte-macrophage colony stimulating factor (GM-CSF) to enhance the immunogenicity of the tumor and to activate antigen-presenting cells.

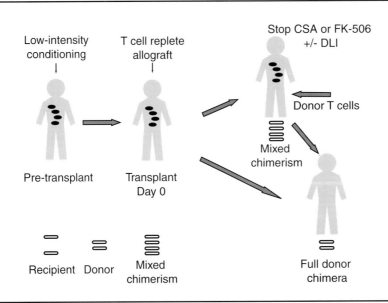

Figure 1. Non-myeloablative transplant approach for solid tumors. Non-myeloablative immunosuppressive conditioning is given to permit the engraftment of donor cells. The conditioning regimen has no direct effect on malignant cells (● = tumor cells). Early chimerism is mixed which protects from GVHD but may also induce a state of tumor tolerance. Following engraftment, T cell chimerism converts to 100% donor, followed by induction of a GVT effect, eradicating all malignant cells. Cyclosporine (CSA) or FK-506 is withdrawn and donor lymphocytes are infused to patients with persistent mixed T cell chimerism or disease progression to enhance an anti-tumor effect.

Advantages of allogeneic immunotherapy over autologous approaches

There are a number of reasons to speculate that allogeneic based immunotherapeutic strategies may be superior to those based on the manipulation of autologous immunity. First, an allograft provides the opportunity to attack the tumor with a chemotherapy naïve donor immune system, which has yet to develop tolerance to tumor antigens. Secondly, patients with growing tumors may lack the T cell repertoire necessary to recognize and destroy the tumor, analogous to what has been observed in patients with leukemia. Finally, over and above the presentation of known tumor specific antigens, malignant cells may present a diversity of allo-antigens to the donor immune system, which could induce powerful anti-tumor responses.[18.]

Stem cell transplants for solid tumors in man

The clinical experience of stem cell allografts in solid tumors is mostly anecdotal. To date, only a few case reports exist where allogeneic lymphocytes have been clearly shown to induce a GVT effect in non-hematologic malignancies. Although murine models have provided some evidence for an allo-immune mediated anti-solid tumor effect,[19] the concern for an unacceptably high risk of transplant-related mortality with conventional allogeneic transplantation has limited the investigation of GVT effects in humans with metastatic tumors. There is, however, some evidence that GVT effects can be induced in patients with metastatic breast carcinoma following allogeneic BMT. In 1996 Eibl *et al.* were the first to report the use of an allogeneic BMT to induce a GVT effect in breast cancer.[20] A woman with extensive metastatic breast cancer underwent an experimental allogeneic BMT receiving stem cells from her HLA-identical sibling. Resolution of liver metastases occurred concomitantly with the onset of severe early acute GVHD. T cells obtained at the time of GVHD showed MHC class I-restricted cytotoxicity against several breast carcinoma cell lines partially matched for MHC class I suggesting the presence of minor histocompatability complex (mHA) on these tumor cells. The clinical course and the *in vitro* results suggested that a GVT effect could exist after allogeneic BMT for breast cancer.

A group of investigators at the M. D. Anderson Cancer Center subsequently evaluated allogeneic peripheral blood stem cell transplantation in 10 women with chemoresponsive metastatic breast cancer.[21] Patients were conditioned with a myeloablative regimen of cyclophosphamide, carmustine and thiotepa and received CSA or FK-506 as GVHD prophylaxis. All patients engrafted with three developing grade ≥ II acute GVHD and four experiencing chronic GVHD. After transplantation, one patient achieved a complete remission, five a partial remission, and four had stable disease. In two patients, metastatic liver lesions were noted to regress in association with skin GVHD following the withdrawal of immunosuppression suggesting a GVT effect. These results showed that allogeneic peripheral blood progenitor cell transplantation is feasible in patients with poor-risk metastatic breast cancer; the regression of tumor associated with GVHD provided some evidence for a possible GVT effect. However, because progression of metastatic breast cancer may be slow, longer follow-up and additional trials will be required to clearly establish a beneficial effect of allotransplantation in this disease.

As no compelling laboratory or clinical evidence exists to support the existence of GVT in most solid tumors, investigators will be required to limit their studies to patients with incurable metastatic tumors, where all treatment options known to prolong survival have been exhausted. As a consequence, survival is likely to be invariably low.

Renal cell carcinoma and metastatic melanoma

Few tumors carry a worse prognosis than metastatic melanoma or renal cell carcinoma (RCC), where median survival in a metastatic setting is in the order of 12–15 months and five-year survival is consistently < 5%.[22,23] A recent study of over 1500 patients with metastatic melanoma showed no improvement in survival over a 22-year time period despite the introduction of a variety of innovative treatments.[24] Chemotherapy is ineffective in the majority of cases and does not prolong survival. However, both malignancies stand out among solid tumors because there is increasing evidence that they may be susceptible to T cell immune responses.[25] Spontaneous regressions, although rare, have been described. Biopsies of spontaneously regressing lesions have been shown to contain tumor infiltrating lymphocytes (TIL) with predominantly CD8+ T cell populations exhibiting MHC class I restricted cytotoxicity against autologous tumor targets.[26–28] Adoptive immunotherapy with *ex-vivo* expanded TILs has been shown to induce tumor regression in some patients with melanoma.[29] Furthermore, unlike most solid tumors, these malignancies are sometimes susceptible to immunomodulator therapy such as IL-2 or interferon alpha where T-cells likely represent the principle effectors. Immunomodulator-based therapy can achieve response rates of 10–20%, with some patients achieving long-term disease free survival.[30–32]

This combination of chemoresistance and the potential to respond to immune-based treatments made us suspect that these tumors might be good targets for a GVT effect following the transplantation of an allogeneic immune system.

The regimen

In 1997, we initiated an experimental protocol at the National Institute of Health in Bethesda to evaluate for GVT effects in metastatic RCC and malignant melanoma. Since high-dose chemotherapy is of little value in the treatment of these malignancies, we chose to use a low intensity, non-myeloablative pre-parative regimen to spare patients the toxicity of dose intensive therapy while providing adequate immunosuppression to allow for the engraftment of donor immune cells. Fludarabine and cyclophosphamide were selected as conditioning agents because of their ability to induce profound immunosuppression with minimal associated toxicity.[33] The protocol is illustrated in Figure 2. The preparative regimen consisted of cyclophosphamide 60 mg/kg on days –7 and –6, followed by fludarabine 25 mg/m² i.v. on days –5 to –1 (FC). CSA was given to prevent graft rejection and as GVHD prophylaxis starting on day –4.

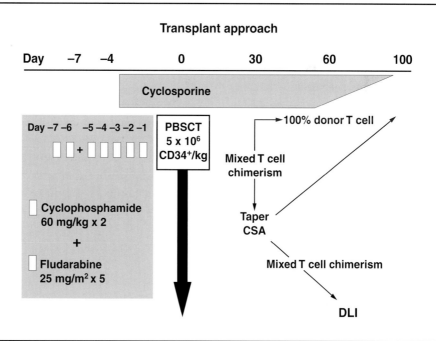

Figure 2. Low intensity transplant protocol. Patients receive conditioning with cyclophosphamide and fludarabine followed by infusion of a G-CSF mobilized peripheral blood stem cell allograft (PBSCT) on day 0. CSA is started on day –4 to prevent graft rejection and continued thereafter as GVHD prophylaxis. Patients with mixed T cell chimerism on day 30 are tapered off CSA and then receive incremental doses of donor lymphocyte infusions (DLI) monthly until GVHD, or disease regression occurs. Patients with 100% donor chimerism by day 30 continue on CSA until day 60 at which point a CSA taper is initiated.

117

HLA identical or single HLA antigen mismatched sibling donors were mobilized with G-CSF (10 μg/kg daily for 5–6 days) with peripheral blood stem cells collected by leukapheresis on day 5, and again on days 6 and 7 if necessary, to achieve a target dose of $\geq 5 \times 10^6$ CD34$^+$ cells/kg of recipient weight.

On day zero, a T cell replete PBSCT containing a high lymphocyte dose (1–4 x 10^8 CD3$^+$/kg) was transfused. To ensure rapid immune recovery, and to maximize the chances of generating a GVT effect, those patients with mixed donor/recipient T-lymphocyte chimerism on day 30 were rapidly tapered off CSA over a 2-week period. Patients not converting to 100% donor chimerism following CSA withdrawal received monthly escalating doses of DLI, with weekly reassessment of chimerism, until 100% donor T cell chimerism, GVHD, or disease regression occurred. In contrast, patients showing 100% donor T-lymphocyte chimerism by day +30 were considered to be at high-risk for the development of acute GVHD and therefore continued full dose CSA until day 60. Thereafter CSA was tapered by 25% every 10 days and discontinued by day 100 if GVHD had not developed. Patients with radiographic evidence of disease progression were rapidly tapered off CSA to enhance an anti-tumor effect. If no GVHD developed, and if tumor progression persisted, patients were eligible for subsequent monthly infusions of incremental doses of DLI as further adoptive anti-tumor immunotherapy.

Patient selection criteria

Eligible patients included adults aged 18–75 years, with biopsy confirmed metastatic melanoma or RCC, which was progressive despite prior cytokine based therapy (with or without chemotherapy) and not amenable to complete surgical resection (Table 1). Patients were required to have either an HLA-identical or single antigen-mismatched sibling donor, and to have radiographically evaluable disease. Patients were excluded for brain metastases, hypercalcemia, or any treatment for their tumor within 30 days of protocol enrollment.

Engraftment

We evaluated the engraftment kinetics in patients with non-hematologic malignancies following NST using PCR analysis of mini-satellite regions on myeloid (CD14$^+$ and CD15$^+$) and T cells (CD3$^+$) which were obtained weekly from peripheral blood samples.[10] A unique pattern of engraftment was observed in which myeloid cells at the time of neutrophil recovery were mixed chimeric, although predominantly recipient in origin in contrast to T cells, which were also mixed chimeric but predominantly donor in origin. By day 30, more than half of the patients had converted to full donor T cell chimerism while myeloid chimerism often remained mixed. Following the withdrawal of CSA,

Table 1. Eligibility criteria for NST in patients with metastatic RCC and melanoma

Protocol eligibility
- Ages 18–75 years
- Biopsy proven metastatic disease, non-amenable to complete surgical resection, progressive despite immunotherapy and/or chemotherapy
- Radiographically evaluable disease
- No prior treatment within 30 days of enrollment
- HLA identical or 5/6 antigen matched family donor
- No evidence of CNS metastatic disease or history of hypercalcemia

and in some patients a DLI, chimerism became complete donor in all cellular lineages in the majority of cases (Figure 3). The establishment of full donor T cell chimerism consistently preceded full donor myeloid chimerism, compatible with a graft-vs-host hematopoiesis effect. Importantly, GVT effects were not observed until full donor T cell chimerism was achieved. T cell chimerism,

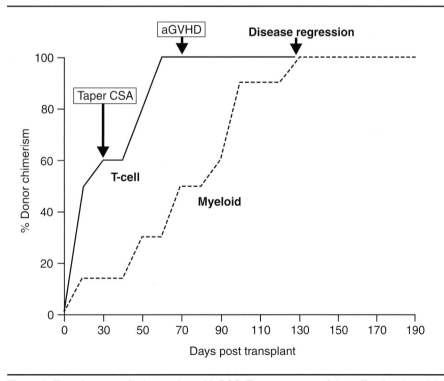

Figure 3. Engraftment profile in a patient with RCC. The percentage of donor T cell and myeloid engraftment at various time-points post-transplant. Donor T cell engraftment (—) and donor myeloid engraftment (– –) are initially mixed. Following tapering of CSA on day 30, T cell chimerism rapidly converts from mixed to 100% donor, followed by the onset of grade II gastrointestinal GVHD which resolves promptly following treatment with methylpredisolone. Myeloid chimerism gradually transitions from mixed to full donor (day 130) consistent with a graft-versus-host hematopoeisis. Disease regression is first noted on computerised tomography (CT) scans by day 130

therefore, appears to be of central importance in terms of outcome following NST and may be used to successfully guide post-transplant immune manipulation.

Toxicity

Despite treating patients with widely metastatic tumors, including several patients with extensive visceral involvement, the regimen was well tolerated. Neutrophil recovery was rapid and occurred at a median of 10 days (range 7–13 days). Mucositis, VOD, and sepsis (bacterial or fungal) did not occur. Acute GVHD grade ≥ II has been the major transplant-related toxicity occurring in 10 (50%) of the first 20 patients treated. The median time to onset of acute GVHD was 45 days (range 28–195 days). GVHD responded to treatment with methylprednisolone and CSA in 9 patients and was fatal in one patient. Four patients developed mild chronic GVHD, three limited to the skin and one in the liver. All 4 responded to low doses of CSA and prednisone.

Clinical evidence for a GVT effect

Although these trials began relatively recently and continue to accrue patients, compelling evidence for the existence of a GVT effect in metastatic RCC has been observed,[34] with five of the first ten patients treated having disease regression, including 2 partial responses and three complete responses. All three patients with a complete response survive without disease progression at 24, 21 and 12 months post-transplant.[35] As of this writing, no clear evidence to support a GVT effect in malignant melanoma has been observed; none of the first eight patients with metastatic melanoma have had a sustained disease response. Although two early partial responses were observed, they were short in duration and most likely reflected a transient response to cyclophosphamide therapy. In contrast, disease regression observed in the patients with metastatic RCC has been durable to date, typically delayed in onset, occurring at a median of 4 months post-transplant following the withdrawal of CSA and establishment of 100% donor T cell chimerism, compatible with a donor mediated GVT effect. A summary of the clinical history and outcome of 2 patients with metastatic RCC treated with NST is given below.

RCC patient # 1

A 50-year-old man developed progressive metastatic disease refractory to alpha interferon treatment seven months after a left nephrectomy for stage III RCC. The patient had an HLA identical sibling and subsequently underwent NST using the above described conditioning regimen. PCR analysis of minisatellites initially showed mixed chimerism in myeloid cells, T-cells and CD34+ progenitor cells, with rapid conversion to 100% donor T cell chimerism by day +60 and 100% myeloid cells by day +110. Serial CT scans of the chest showed stable disease at day +30, slight regression of pulmonary lesions at day +63, and complete disappearance of all pulmonary metastatic disease by day +110 (Figure 4). Multiple bone metastases were noted to have regressed completely by follow-up bone scan on day 203.

Analysis of lymphoid subsets at the time of disease regression revealed a significant increase in the percentage of activated cytotoxic T lymphocytes (from 7% to 47 % HLA-DR positive) with a decrease in the percentage of natural killer cells (CD3$^-$, CD2$^+$, CD16$^+$, CD56$^+$) compatible with a donor T-cell mediated anti-tumor response. The patient subsequently returned to work following transplantation and remains in remission more than 2 years post-transplant.

RCC patient # 2

A 48-year-old male was found to have an 8 x 8 cm right renal mass following a work-up for flank pain and hematuria. Eight months after a radical nephrectomy he developed extensive pulmonary metastasis, as well as recurrent disease in his right renal fossa. Treatment with IL-2 and interferon alpha was unsuccessful, and he subsequently underwent NST from his HLA-identical brother. Engraftment was rapid with 100% donor T-cell chimerism documented 21 days post-transplant. Acute GVHD of the gastrointestinal tract (Grade II) occurred on day 32 and responded promptly to treatment with methylprednisolone (1 mg/kg/day). Day 60 and day 100 CT scans revealed progression of metastatic disease. CSA was tapered off by day 100, with follow-up CT scans on day 130 revealing a dramatic regression in all metastatic lesions. By day 220, pulmonary metastatic disease had completely resolved and retroperitoneal lymphadenopathy had regressed by > 75%. The patient continues to do well 18 months post-transplant with minimal and stable retroperitoneal disease.

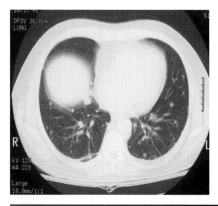 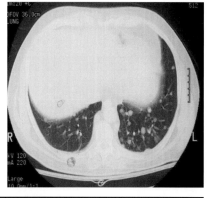

Figure 4a. Baseline CT images of a patient with RCC with widely metastatic pulmonary disease. A biopsy of the lung nodule confirms metastatic disease (clear cell histology).

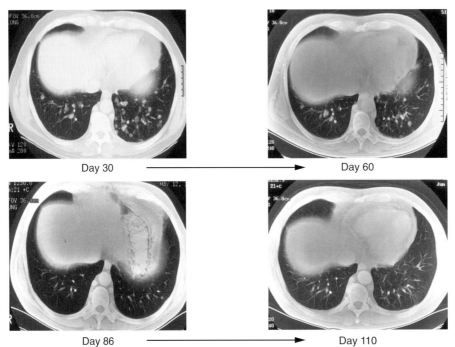

Day 30 ⟶ Day 60

Day 86 ⟶ Day 110

Figure 4b. Serial images of a single CT reveals no change in disease at day 30, regression of pulmonary nodules beginning at day 60, followed by rapid and complete regression of all disease by day 110

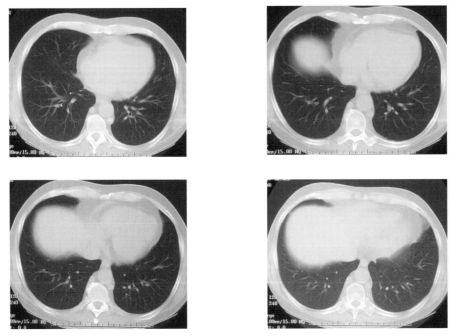

Figure 4c. CT images 2 years post-transplant showing persistent remission of disease

122

In summary

These preliminary results provide some of the first evidence that NST can be carried out safely in patients with advanced metastatic solid tumors, and that GVT effects resulting in complete regression of disease can be achieved. Furthermore, the disease responses in RCC following this approach seem durable, and were achieved in patients who had failed to respond to conventional immune-based strategies. Evidence indicates that the anti-tumor effects observed in RCC were mediated through allogeneic T cells. Disease regressions occurred only after full donor T cell chimerism was achieved and usually were not observed until CSA had been completely withdrawn. Furthermore, the interval from transplant conditioning to disease regression was prolonged (median 4 months), a time pattern analogous to patients receiving lymphocyte transfusions to treat relapsed chronic myelogenous leukemia. This prolonged interval to disease regression probably represents the time required for the proliferation and expansion of a relatively small population of tumor reactive T-cells contained within the allograft.

The high response rate observed in this trial provides the opportunity for the expansion and cloning of tumor specific T-cells for the identification and characterization of candidate tumor antigens. Once identified, these antigens could be used for the *in-vitro* expansion of tumor specific CTL to be infused concomitantly with the allograft. Such a targeted approach might shorten the interval to a disease response and could enhance the overall efficacy of this treatment approach.

The patients who failed conventional cytokine-based immunotherapy and subsequently responded to NST provide evidence that adoptive allogeneic immunotherapy may be more potent than strategies designed to enhance autologous anti-tumor immunity. It is, therefore, likely that increasing numbers of investigators will attempt allogeneic stem cell transplants in a widening variety of tumors. Because animal models have usually not proven to be predictive in humans, tumor-specific investigations will be required to establish the existence of GVT effects in other refractory malignancies.

References

1. Weiden P, Flournoy N, Thomas E, Prentice R, Fefer A, Buckner CD, Storb R. Antileukemic effects of graft-versus-host disease in human recipients of allogeneic marrow grafts. *New Engl J Med* 1979; 300: 1068–73.

2. Sosman JA, Sondel PM. The graft versus leukemia effect following bone marrow transplantation: A review of laboratory and clinical data. *Hematol Rev* 1987; 2: 77.

3. Horowitz M, Gale RP, Sondel P, Goldman JM, Kersey J, Kolb HJ, Rimm AA, Ringden O, Rozman C, Speck B. Graft-versus-leukemia reactions after bone marrow transplantation. *Blood* 1990; 75: 555–62.

4. Offit K, Burns JP, Cunningham I, Jhanwar SC, Black P, Kernan NA, O'Reilly RJ, Chaganti RSK. Cytogenetic analysis of chimerism and leukemia relapse in chronic myelogenous leukemia patients after T-cell depleted bone marrow transplantation. *Blood* 1990; 75: 1346–55.

5. Marmont AM, Horowitz MM, Gale RP, Sobocinski K, Ash RC, van Bekkum DW, Champlin RE, Dicke KA, Goldman JM, Good RA. T-cell depletion of HLA-identical transplants in leukemia. *Blood* 1991; 78: 2120–30.

6. Kolb HJ, Mittermueller J, Clemm C Holler E, Ledderose G, Brehm G, Heim M, Wilmanns W. Donor leukocyte transfusions for treatment of recurrent chronic myelogenous leukemia in marrow transplant patients. *Blood* 1990; 76: 2462–65.

7. Drobyski WR, Keever CA, Roth MS, Koethe S. Hanson G, McFadden P, Gottschall JR, Ash RC, van Tuinen P, Horowitz MM, Flomenberg N. Salvage immunotherapy using donor leukocyte infusions as treatment for relapsed chronic myelogenous leukemia after bone marrow transplantation: Efficacy and toxicity of a defined T-cell dose. *Blood* 1993; 82: 2310–18.

8. Giralt S, Estey E, Albitar M, van Besien K, Rondon G, Anderlini P, O'Brien S, Khouri I, Gajewski J, Mehra R, Claxton D, Andersson B, Beran M, Przepiorka D, Koller C, Kornblau S, Korbling M, Keating M, Kantarjian H, Champlin R. Engraftment of allogeneic hematopoietic progenitor cells with purine analog containing chemotherapy: Harnessing graft-versus-leukemia without myeloablative therapy. *Blood* 1997; 89: 4531–6.

9. Slavin S, Nagler A, Naparstek E Kapelushnik Y, Aker M, Cividalli G, Varadi G, Kirschbaum M, Ackerstein A, Samuel S, Amar A, Brautbar C, Ben-Tal O, Eldor A, Or R. Non-myeloablative stem cell transplantation and cell therapy as an alternative to conventional bone marrow transplantation with lethal cytoreduction for the treatment of malignant and nonmalignant hematological diseases. *Blood* 1998; 91: 756–63.

10. Childs R, Clave E, Contentin N Jayasekera D, Hensel N, Leitman S, Read EJ, Carter C, Bahceci E, Young NS, Barrett AJ. Engraftment kinetics after nonmyeloablative allogeneic peripheral blood stem cell transplantation: Full donor T-cell chimerism precedes alloimmune responses. *Blood* 1999; 94: 3234–41.

11. Sykes M, Preffer F, McAfee S, Saidman SL, Weymouth D, Andrews DM, Colby C, Sackstein R, Sachs DH, Spitzer TR. Mixed lymphohaemopoietic chimerism and graft-versus-lymphoma effects after non-myeloablative therapy and HLA mismatched bone-marrow transplantation. *Lancet* 1999; 353: 1755–59.

12. Childs R, Epperson D, Bahceci E, Clave E, Barrett J. Molecular remission of chronic myeloid leukaemia following a non-myeloablative allogeneic peripheral blood stem cell transplant: *in vivo* and *in vitro* evidence for a graft-versus-leukaemia effect. *Br J Haematol* 1999; 107: 396–400.

13. Khouri IF, Keating M, Korbling M, Przepiorka D, Anderlini P, O'Brien S, Giralt S, Ippoliti C, von Wolff B, Gajewski J, Donato M, Claxton D, Ueno N, Andersson B, Gee A, Champlin R. Transplant-lite: induction of graft-versus-malignancy using fludarabine-based nonablative chemotherapy and allogeneic blood progenitor-cell transplantation as a treatment for lymphoid malignancies. *J Clin Oncol* 1998; 18: 2817–24.

14. Gattoni-Celli S, Kirsch K, Timpane R, Isselbacher KJ. Beta 2 microglobulin is mutated in human colon cancer cell line deficient in the expression of HLA class I antigens on the cell surface. *Cancer Res* 1992; 52: 1201–04.

15. Rivoltini L, Barracchini K, Viggiano V, Kawakami Y, Smith A, Mixon A, Restifo NP, Topalian SL, Simonis TB, Rosenberg SA. Quantitative correlation between HLA class I expression and recognition of melanoma cells by antigen-specific T lymphocytes. *Cancer Res* 1995; 55: 3149–57.

16. Hahne M, Rimoldi D, Schroter M, Romero P, Schreier M, French LE, Schneider P, Bornand T, Fontana A, Lienard D, Cerottini J, Tschopp J. Melanoma cell expression of Fas ligand: Implications of tumor escape. *Science* 1996; 274: 1363–6.

17. Huber D, Phillip J, Fontana A. Protease inhibitors interfere with TGF-beta dependent pathway of tumor cell mediated immunosuppression. *J Immunol* 1992; 148: 277–84.

18. Mukherji B, Chakraborty NG. Immunobiology and immunotherapy of melanoma. *Curr Opin Oncol* 1995; 7: 175–84.

19. Morecki S; Moshel Y; Gelfend Y, Pugatsch T, Slavin S. Induction of graft vs. tumor effect in a murine mammary adenocarcinoma. *Int J Cancer* 1997; 71(1): 59–63.

20. Eibl B, Schwaighofer H, Nachbaur D, Marth C, Gachter A, Knapp R, Bock G, Gassner C, Schiller L, Petersen F, Niederwieser D. Evidence of a graft-versus-tumor effect in a patient treated with marrow ablative chemotherapy and allogeneic bone marrow transplantation for breast cancer. *Blood* 1996; 88: 1501–8.

21. Ueno NT, Rondon G, Mirza NQ, Geisler DK, Anderlini P, Giralt SA, Andersson BS, Claxton DF, Gajewski JL, Khouri IF, Korbling M, Mehra RC, Przepiorka D, Rahman Z, Samuels BI, van Besien K, Hortobagyi GN, Champlin RE. Allogeneic peripheral-blood progenitor-cell transplantation for poor-risk patients with metastatic breast cancer. *J Clin Oncol* 1998; 16: 986–93.

22. Houghton AN, Meyers ML, Chapman PB. Medical treatment of metastatic melanoma. *Surg Clin North Am* 1996; 76: 1343–53.

23. Elson PJ, Witte RS, Trump DI. Prognostic factors for survival in patients with recurrent or metastatic renal cell carcinoma. *Cancer Res* 1988; 48: 7310–13.

24. Barth A, Wanek LA, Morton D. Prognostic factors in 1,521 melanoma patients with distant metastases. *J Am Coll Surg* 1995; 181: 193–201.

25. Mukherji B, Chakraborty NG. Immunobiology and immunotherapy of melanoma. *Curr Opin Oncol* 1995; 7: 175–84.

26. Halliday GM, Patel A, Hunt M, Tefany FJ, Barnetson RS. Spontaneous regression of human melanoma/nonmelanoma skin cancer: Association with infiltrating CD4+ T cells. *World J Surg* 1995; 19: 352–8.

27. Melioli G, Guastella M, Semino C, Meta M, Pietra G, Ponte M, Queirolo P, Sertoli MR, Martini L, Reali UM. Proliferative, phenotypic and functional and molecular characteristics of tumor-infiltrating lymphocytes obtained from unselected patients with malignant melanomas and expanded in vitro in the presence of recombinant interleukin-2. *Melanoma Res* 1994; 4: 127–33.

28. Topalian SL, Solomon D, Avis FP, Chang AE, Freerksen DL, Linehan WM, Lotze MT, Robertson CN, Seipp CA, Simon P. Immunotherapy of patients with advanced cancer using tumor-infiltrating lymphocytes and recombinant interleukin-2. A pilot study. *J Clin Oncol* 1988; 6: 839–53.

29. Kradin RL, Kurnick JT, Lazarus DS, Preffer FI, Dubinett SM, Pinto CE, Gifford J, Davidson E, Grove B, Callahan RJ. Tumor-infiltrating lymphocytes and interleukein-2 in treatment of advanced cancer. *Lancet* 1989;1: 577–80.

30. Rosenberg SA, Yang JC, Topalian SL, Schwartzentruber DJ, Weber JS, Parkinson DR, Seipp CA, Einhorn JH, White DE. Treatment of 283 consecutive patients with metastatic melanoma or renal cell carcinoma using high-dose bolus interleukin 2. *JAMA* 1994; 271: 907–13.

31. Gleave ME, Elhilali M, Fradet Y, Davis I, Venner P, Saad F, Klotz LH, Moore MJ, Paton V, Bajamonde A. Interferon gamma-1b compared to placebo in metastatic renal-cell carcinoma. *N Engl J Med* 1998; 338: 1265–71.

32. Negrier S, Escudier B, Lasset C, Douillard JY, Savary J, Chevreau C, Ravaud A, Mercatello A, Peny J, Mousseau M, Philip T, Tursz T. Recombinant human interleukin-2, recombinant human interferon alfa 2a, or both in metastatic renal-cell carcinoma. *N Engl J Med* 1998; 1272–78.

33. Plunkett W, Sanders PP. Metabolism and action of purine nucleoside analogs. *Pharmacol Ther* 1991; 49: 239–68.

34. Childs R, Clave E, Tisdale J, Plante M, Hensel N, Barrett J. Successful treatment of metastatic renal cell carcinoma with a non-myeloablative allogeneic peripheral blood progenitor cell transplant: Evidence for a graft-versus-tumor effect. *J Clin Oncol* 1999; 17: 2044–51.

35. Childs R. Contentin N, Clave E, Bahceci E, Chernoff A, Linehan M, Epperson D, Jayasekera D, Eniafe R, Young NS, Barrett AJ. Sustained regression of metastatic renal cell carcinoma following nonmyeloablative allogeneic peripheral blood stem transplantation. A new application of allogeneic immunotherapy. *Blood* 1999; 94: 710a.

Non-myeloablative stem cell transplantation for non-malignant disorders

R Or, M Aker, A Nagler, S Slavin

Introduction

High-dose chemotherapy followed by allogeneic bone marrow transplantation (BMT) is the preferred treatment for many non-malignant hematologic diseases, including thalassemia major (TM).[1–3] The pre-transplant chemotherapy has a 2-fold purpose, namely to destroy hematopoietic host cells in order to gain marrow space and, concomitantly, to induce adequate immunosuppression in an attempt to prevent rejection of donor stem cells.

Despite the significant and ongoing improvements in conditioning regimens used for allogeneic BMT, patients may ultimately develop either persistent host lymphohematopoietic cells or their underlying disease will relapse. Various studies have demonstrated that patients who are in good clinical condition after BMT and have normal hematologic parameters may still harbor minimal amounts of residual host hematopoietic cells in their bone marrow and peripheral blood.[4–6] The methods used to detect chimerism post-BMT for non-malignant disorders include detection of sex chromosomes in cases of sex disparity between donor and recipient,[7] analysis of hypervariable regions of the human genome by polymerase chain reaction (PCR) amplification[4,7–11] and ABO typing.[12]

We used the detection of point mutation in the β-globin gene as a measure of outcome in patients with TM undergoing BMT. This innovative technique provides the means of establishing the degree of chimerism, and allows correlation between the degree of chimerism and the clinical outcome post-BMT. To illustrate the validity and practical usefulness of this technique, results from a series of 20 evaluable patients (out of 35 consecutive thalassemia patients) who received a BMT and in whom β-globin gene point mutation was analyzed will be discussed, although these patients were treated with conventional BMT using standard rather than fludarabine-containing regimens. We will also present two detailed case reports.

Chimerism post-BMT in patients with TM

Twenty patients (median age = 29 months, range = 9 months to 7 years,) with TM were treated with BMT at our institution during an 11-year period (1984–1995). All patients received allogeneic BMT from human leukocyte antigen (HLA)-identical, related donors. Eight of the 20 donor–recipient pairs were sex-mismatched. Patients received oral busulfan (4 mg/kg x 4 days) and intravenous cyclophosphamide (50 mg/kg x 4 days). Thiotepa (5 mg/kg x 1 day) was added to the regimen in 14 patients. *In vivo* depletion of host lymphocytes prior to chemotherapy was achieved using total lymphoid irradiation ([TLI] 1000 cGy given in 5 daily fractions) in 21 patients and i.v. rat anti-human CD52 (IgG2b) antibody (CAMPATH-1G 0.2 mg/kg x 4 days) in 14 patients.

Graft-versus-host disease prophylaxis consisted of CAMPATH-1M used *in vitro* with donor serum as the source of complement (*n* = 21) or CAMPATH-1G used *ex vivo* directly into the bone marrow collection bag (*n* = 14) to produce T cell depleted (TCD) marrow.[13–16] Cyclosporine A (CSA) (3 mg/kg/day i.v.) was given to all patients from day 1 to engraftment (number of polymorphonuclear cells $\geq 750/mm^2$) to prevent rejection. DNA was prepared from peripheral blood according to standard procedures.[17] PCR was carried out using Taq polymerase in the 20 evaluable patients.

Following BMT, peripheral blood samples were analyzed sequentially for detection of the β-globin gene point mutations. Six patients (30%) were found to have full engraftment (100% donor cells) and currently these patients are in excellent clinical condition, exhibiting normal growth and development; their hemoglobin (Hb) levels are comparable with those of their respective donors. Mixed chimerism was detected in 11 (55%) patients, 10 of whom have 70–96% donor cells with stable mixed chimerism; they are independent of blood transfusions, and are in excellent clinical condition. The eleventh patient has 4–7% donor cells with only a minimal transfusion requirement; she presents clinically with thalassemia intermedia. The remaining three patients (15%) have no detectable donor genes (i.e. 100% host cells) and have persistent TM.

The 10 patients with 70–96% donor cells have red blood cell (RBC) counts similar to those of their donors; the stable mixed chimerism in this group of patients indicates sustained engraftment with no recurrence of the underlying disease. None of the 20 patients showed signs of acute or chronic GVHD. To date, the period of follow up and clinical investigation ranges between 3.5 and 15 years (median 7.5 years). The clinical course of two TM patients will be presented in detail.

Patient 1

An 18-month-old female with β-TM underwent an allogeneic BMT in February 1988 from her HLA-matched mixed lymphocyte culture (MLC) non-reactive grandmother. There was a major ABO mismatch (A$^+$ → O$^+$). The conditioning regimen consisted of TLI (2 cGy x 4 days) followed by busulfan (16 mg/kg) and cyclophosphamide (200 mg/kg). *In vitro* TCD of the marrow was accomplished with CAMPATH-1M.[16,19] No post-grafting immunosuppressive GVHD prophylaxis was given. The patient engrafted rapidly and had normal blood counts on day +29.[18]

Fourteen months post-BMT the hemoglobin count (Hb) dropped to 5.7–7.0 g/dL and mean corpuscular volume (MCV) 70–72 fL. A PCR-VNTR (variable number of tandem repeats) test failed to show the presence of donor cells 24, 29, 45 and 51 months post-BMT, whereas the β-globin gene point mutation analysis[20,21] detected 4–7% donor-derived DNA cells. The patient was homozygous for the mutation IVS1, 110/VS1, 110, while the donor was heterozygous for the same mutation. The β-globin assay on cultured erythroid colonies with or without erythropoietin resulted in 16% and 7% donor cells, respectively. Blood group analyses revealed the presence of donor red blood cells (RBC) (Type A). Notwithstanding the mixed chimeric minimal donor cell state, the clinical picture presented as thalassemia intermedia with low transfusion requirements.

Because of the presence of stable mixed chimerism, it was decided to carry out a second ambulatory transplant from the original donor using non-myeloablative conditioning. In August 1994, the patient received oral hydroxyurea (1500 mg/day x 6) followed by an i.v. cyclophosphamide bolus (750 mg). The patient was transplanted with non-manipulated allogeneic peripheral blood stem cells (PBSC) mobilized by subcutaneous injections of granulocyte colony stimulating factor (G-CSF; Neupogen 10 mg/kg/day x 5). The inoculum consisted of 8.74 x 10^8/kg nucleated cells (30.6 x 10^6 CD34$^+$ cells) collected in three successive aphereses on days 4, 5, and 6 after the first injection of G-CSF. No post-transplant immunosuppressive treatment was given. The patient tolerated the procedure well, with no severe neutropenia or thrombocytopenia. A spontaneous increase in Hb level concomitant with a gradual increase in the percentage of donor-derived cells ensued. On day +52 the patient displayed signs of acute GVHD (grade II), involving skin and intestine which was treated with methylprednisone and CSA with good response.

To date 5 years after the second transplant, the patient maintains an Hb count of 12.5 g/dL and excellent clinical performance (Karnofsky performance status of 100%). The donor-specific markers and blood group type, analyzed in

129

the peripheral blood and in marrow aspirates, show 100% reconstitution with donor cells.

Patient 2

A $5\frac{1}{2}$-year-old boy had been diagnosed with β-TM at the age of 3+ months. The patient had been transfused monthly without chelation therapy for nine months prior to BMT. His Hb level was 6.1 g/dL; direct and indirect agglutination tests were positive for the red cell antigens Kell and E. Gross hyperplasia of the maxillary bone, typical of poorly controlled β-TM, was evident. The spleen was enlarged and palpable 6 cm below the left costal margin.

The pre-BMT conditioning regimen included oral busulfan (4 mg/kg/day x 1) followed by cyclophosphamide i.v. (50 mg/kg/day x 4). Prior to chemotherapy, the patient was treated with monoclonal rat anti-human CD52 antibody (CAMPATH-1G, 0.2 mg/kg/day x 4). In April 1991, the patient underwent an allogeneic TCD BMT from a fully HLA-matched sister. Both patient and donor were blood group O[+].[22] CAMPATH-1G was added to the bone marrow collection bag (0.3 mg/10^6 nucleated cells). The inoculum contained 5 x 10^8 nucleated cells/kg. A maintenance course of CSA (3 mg/kg/day) was given to prevent rejection until tri-lineage engraftment was confirmed, after which the drug was tapered off (at day +36). G-CSF (5 mg/kg/day) was given from day +1 until neutrophil counts were 0.5 x 10^9/L on two consecutive days.

The conditioning regimen was well tolerated. Total white blood cell (WBC) nadir occurred on day +5, an absolute granulocyte count of 0.5 x 10^9/L was reached on day +14 and an unsupported platelet count of 50 x 10^9/L was reached on day +36. GVHD did not develop and the patient was discharged on day +27 in good clinical condition.

The sex chromosomes in the marrow and in peripheral blood lymphocytes (PBL) were analyzed as engraftment markers using standard cytogenetic and PCR analysis techniques for the detection of X- and Y-specific amelogenin gene (AMG-PCR). AMG-PCR of genomic DNA from PBL on day +61 showed the typical pattern of a mixed chimerism with about 30% male residual host cells. In parallel, the cytogenetic analysis of spontaneously dividing marrow cells showed only 71% donor (female) cells. In an attempt to prevent recurrence of the underlying disease, a donor lymphocyte infusion (DLI) was given to eradicate residual host-derived stem cells. Graded increments of donor T cells, obtained by leukopheresis without growth factor stimulation, were infused, starting with 10^5 cells/kg on day +84. On day +97 cytogenetic analysis of phytohemagglutinin-responding PBL showed 65% host-type cells, and an analysis of spontaneously dividing marrow cells revealed 20% host-derived cells. In the absence of GVHD, a second infusion of 5 x 10^7 donor T cells/kg obtained without G-CSF was administered on day +98. Three weeks later, 27% of phytohemagglutinin-responsive cells in the PBL were still of male (recipient) karyotype. The patient remained reticulocytopenic and continued to be dependent on transfusions of RBC and platelets; WBC counts, on the other hand, were normal with 70% granulocytes. An acute hemolytic disorder that developed in association with panagglutinins for RBC (positive direct agglutination test) responded to a two-week course of steroid therapy. There was no clinical or biochemical evidence of GVHD. On day +136 an additional bolus of 2.5 x 10^7 donor T cells/kg (collected by leukopheresis without G-CSF) was given. During the next eight weeks, transfusion requirements diminished along with progressive reticulocytosis, and the direct agglutinin test became negative. On day +235, the patient showed signs of acute GVHD (grade II) involving the oral cavity, which responded to short-term treatment with corticosteroids and CSA. By day +242, there was engraftment with 100% donor-derived cells; both the AMG-PCR and the β-globin gene mutation test confirmed full donor chimerism.

Several conclusions can be drawn from our experience using allogeneic BMT in patients with β-TM. The incidence of mixed chimerism was higher than was expected from published studies, which led us to surmise that post-transplant mixed chimerism in non-malignant diseases is under reported. The conditioning regimen, manipulation of the graft, and the mode of GVHD prophylaxis may play a crucial role in the induction of stable mixed chimerism.[24–26] In addition, the role of post-transplant DLI as cell-mediated immunotherapy for the elimination of residual host cells in patients with non-malignant diseases still required clarification.[27,28] Our findings in TM patients imply that total eradication of the host hematopoietic system to ensure sustained engraftment is not an absolute necessity.

Fludarabine-containing preparatory regimens

Based on our results with non-myeloablative regimens in malignant hematologic diseases,[24] we gave fludarabine-containing conditioning regimens to patients with a variety of non-malignant stem cell-dependent diseases prior to allogeneic BMT. The disorders comprised thalassemia ($n = 6$), severe aplastic anemia ($n = 5$), Fanconi's anemia ($n = 3$), osteopetrosis ($n = 2$) chronic granulomatous disease (CGD) ($n = 2$), combined immunodeficiency (CID) ($n = 1$), Blackfan Diamond syndrome ($n = 1$) and Gaucher's disease ($n = 1$). All patients were transplanted from fully HLA-matched related donors. The particular nature of the different diseases, the widely diverging ages of the patients, and the fact that the setting was that of a pilot study, forced variations in the preparatory regimens, however all regimens included fludarabine.[25,26,29,30]

The basic NST protocol consists of intensive immunosuppression with fludarabine (30 mg/m^2 days –10 to –5), anti-T lymphocyte globulin (ATG) (Fresenius, 5–10 mg/kg days –4 to –1), and mild cytoreduction with oral busulfan (4 mg/kg on days –6 and –5).[24]

Blackfan Diamond syndrome
This protocol was used in a 31-year-old female patient with Blackfan Diamond syndrome. Prior to the NST (which was carried out on November 27, 1996) the patient had received more than 500 blood transfusions. Following NST, she displayed rapid engraftment with 100% donor cells. She experienced acute and chronic GVHD, which responded to steroid therapy. Fourteen months after the transplant she succumbed to overwhelming pneumococcal infection.

Gaucher's disease
The same basic NST protocol was used to treat a 3-year-old female with Gaucher's disease who was transplanted on January 27, 1997. There was full engraftment and, to date, the patient has normal growth and development.

β-TM
A 24-year-old female who had received over 800 blood transfusions received an NST on August 25, 1999. Since this was a high-risk patient a single dose of 200 cGy total body irradiation (TBI) was added to the conditioning regimen. The patient had full engraftment with concomitant grade IV GVHD, which was resolved with immunosuppressive therapy. Currently, she has 100% Karnofsky score and enjoys a normal life.

The results of patients with β-TM treated with NST are shown in Table 1. The dose of busulphan was altered for pediatric patients with TM (total dose given was 16 mg/kg) to take account of its pharmacokinetics.

Severe aplastic anemia
For patients with severe aplastic anemia optimal immunosuppression rather than myeloablation is required. We therefore substituted cyclophosphamide (60 mg/kg/day) for busulfan in the basic NST protocol. As shown in Table 2, in each of these five high-risk patients the transplant course was uncomplicated, without manifestations of GVHD, and the outcome was satisfactory.

Table 1. NST for β-TM – patient characteristics and outcome

Patient number	Age (years)	Date of BMT	Engraftment	GVHD	Survival
1057[1]	6	4.7.96	+	–	a & w
1194[1]	12	30.7.97	+	–	a & w
1311	6	29.7.98	+ → –	–	a & w/tm
1390[2]	4	10.3.99	+ → –	–	a & w/tm
1455[1]	6	3.11.99	+	+	a & w
1436[3]	24	25.8.99	+	+	a & w

[1] Conditioned with busulfan 4 mg/kg/day x 4
[2] DLI induced aplasia; reconstitution with host cells
[3] Conditioned with fludarabine 30 mg/m²/day x 6 and TBI 200 cGy

Table 2. NST for severe aplastic anemia– patient characteristics and outcome

Patient number	Age (years)	Prior ATG	Date of BMT	Engraftment	GVHD	Survival (months)
1228	12	+	6.11.97	+	–	26
1267	42	+	11.7.98	+	–	20
1281	26	–	20.4.98	+	–	21
1293	9	–	1.6.98	+	–	19
1445	13	–	21.9.99	+	–	4

Fanconi's anemia

Patients with Fanconi's anemia do not tolerate aggressive conditioning because of genetically determined ineffective DNA repair. The NST protocol was therefore changed even more radically such that fludarabine was given for 5 days and the dose of cyclophosphamide was lowered to 10 mg/kg/day.[31] The treatment resulted in an excellent outcome in all three patients (Table 3).

Table 3. NST for Fanconi's anemia – patient characteristics and outcome

Patient number	Age (years)	Date of BMT	Engraftment	GVHD	Survival (months)
1114	10	10.10.96	+	–	38
1202	12	17.8.97	+	–	29
1420	10	23.6.99	+	+	7

Other genetic disorders

Two infant patients with osteopetrosis received a modified NST protocol (busulfan 16 mg/kg, total dose) that resulted in durable engraftment and good outcome (Table 4). One of the two patients with CGD, a 39-year-old male who required oxygen support 24 hours a day, received TBI (a single dose of 200 cGy) subsequent to administration of fludarabine. The patient converted to full donor chimerism, experiencing only mild GVHD. His neutrophil function test normalized with no manifestations of infectious episodes. The pulmonary function tests are continually improving, and to date he requires minimal oxygen assistance for limited periods of time, enabling him to go out of the house and walk about freely.

Table 4. NST for other genetic diseases – patient characteristics and outcome

Patient number	Age	Disease	BMT	Engraftment	GVHD	Survival
1139	6 years	CGD	21.1.97	+	–	a & w
1277[1]	2 months	ostepetrosis	9.4.98	+	–	a & w
1317[1]	5 months	ostepetrosis	12.8.98	+	–	a & w
1400[2]	39 years	CGD	27.4.99	+	+	a & w
1441[2]	11 years	CID	9.9.99	+	+	died 8 months post-NST

[1]Conditioned with busulfan 4 mg/kg/day x 4
[2]Conditioned with fludarabine 30 mg/m² x 6 and TBI 200 cGy

Graft-versus autoimmune disease[32,33]

A 37-year-old male patient with chronic myeloid leukemia in chronic phase also had severe cutaneous psoriasis and psoriatic arthritis. On January 29, 1997 he underwent the basic NST protocol, using his HLA-matched sister as donor. One month post-transplant engraftment markers revealed mixed chimerism in conjunction with active skin psoriasis on the forehead, chest, neck and elbows; polyarthritis especially in the interphalangeal joints of both hands was also noted. In order to exploit the alloreactive potential of the donor T cells with the aim of inducing both graft-versus-leukemia and graft-versus-autoimmune disease reactions, CSA treatment was stopped; 46 days later GVHD grade II was observed. Concurrent with the development of GVHD, the psoriatic signs and symptoms resolved completely. Chimeric studies recently revealed showed 100% donor chimerism; currently the patient has no signs of leukemia or psoriasis.

In summary

The non-myeloablative protocol designed for the treatment of malignant diseases constituted the basis of our therapeutic approach to various non-malignant disorders. The ability to achieve engraftment with non-ablative regimens means that it is now possible to segregate the elements directed at the eradication of leukemia and those that aim at induction of immunoablation. The fludarabine-based NST protocol with its disease-specific modifications as detailed here, allowed engraftment with minimal toxicity in a variety of genetic and non-malignant life-threatening diseases.

References

1. Lucarelli G, Galimberti M, Polchi P, Angelucci E, Baronciani D, Giardini C, Politi P, Durazzi SM, Muretto P, Albertini F. Bone marrow transplantation in patients with thalassemia. *N Engl J Med* 1990; 322: 417–21.

2. Lucarelli G, Galimberti M, Polchi P, Angelucci E, Baronciani D, Giardini C, Andreani M, Agostinelli F, Albertini F, Clift RA. Marrow transplantation in patients with thalassemia responsive to iron chelation therapy. *N Engl J Med* 1993; 329: 840–4.

3. Rund D, Rachmilewitz E. Advances in the pathophysiology and treatment of thalassemia. *Critical Rev Oncol Hematol* 1995; 20: 237–54.

4. Lawler M, Humphries P, McCann SR. Evaluation of mixed chimerism by *in vitro* amplification of dinucleotide repeat sequences using the polymerase chain reaction. *Blood* 1991; 77: 2504–14.

5. Manna M, Nesci S, Andreani M, Tonucci P, Lucarelli G. Influence of the conditioning regimens on the incidence of mixed chimerism in thalassemia transplanted patients. *Bone Marrow Transplant* 1993; 12 (Suppl. 1): 70–3.

6. Nesci S, Manna M, Andreani M, Fattorini P, Graziosi G, Lucarelli G. Mixed chimerism in thalassemic patients after bone marrow transplantation. *Bone Marrow Transplant* 1992; 10: 143–6.

7. Durnam DM, Anders KR, Fisher L, O'Quigley J, Bryant EM, Thomas ED. Analysis of the origin of marrow cells in the bone marrow transplant recipients using a Y-chromosome-specific in situ hybridization assay. *Blood* 1989; 74: 2220–6.

8. Blazar BR, Orr HT, Arthur DC, Kersey JH, Fillipovich AH. Restriction fragment length polymorphism as markers of engraftment in allogeneic marrow transplantation. *Blood* 1985; 66: 1436–44.

9. Chalmers EA, Sproul AM, Mills KI, Gibson BE, Burnett AK. Use of the polymerase chain reaction to monitor engraftment following allogeneic bone marrow transplantation. *Bone Marrow Transplant* 1990; 6: 399–403.

10. Roth MS, Antin JH, Bingham EL, Ginsburg D. Use of polymerase chain reaction-detected sequence polymorphism to document engraftment following allogeneic bone marrow transplantation. *Transplantation* 1990; 49: 714–20.

11. Uggozoli L, Yam P, Petz LD, Ferrara GB, Champlin RE, Forman SJ, Koyal D, Wallace RB. Amplification by the polymerase chain reaction of hypervariable regions of the human genome for evaluation of chimerism after bone marrow transplantation. *Blood* 1991;77: 1607–15.

12. Bar BM, Schattenberg A, van Dijk BA, de Man AJM, Kunst VAJM, de Winter T. Host and donor erythrocyte repopulation patterns after allogeneic bone marrow transplantation analysed with antibody-coated fluorescent microspheres. *Br J Haematol* 1989; 72: 239–45.

13. Cobbold S, Martin G, Waldmann H. Monoclonal antibodies for the prevention of graft versus host disease and marrow graft rejection. The depletion of T cell subsets *in vitro* and *in vivo*. *Transplantation* 1986; 42: 239–47.

14. Naparstek E, Hardan L, Ben-Shahar H, *et al*. A new method for prevention of graft versus host disease (GVHD). Proceedings from the XVIII Annual Meeting of the International Society for Experimental Hematology, Paris, France, 1989, p. 723 (abstract 17).

15. Slavin S, Waldmann H, Or R, *et al*. Prevention of graft vs host disease in allogeneic bone marrow transplantation for leukemia by T cell depletion *in vitro* prior to transplantation. *Transplant Proc* 1985; 17: 465–7.

16. Waldmann H, Polliak A, Hale G, Or R, Cividalli G, Weiss L, Weshler Z, Samuel S, Manor D, Brautbar C. Elimination of graft-versus-host disease by *in vivo* depletion of alloreactive lymphocytes with a monoclonal rat anti human lymphocyte antibody (CAMPATH-1). *Lancet* 1984; 2: 482–6.

17. Miller SA, Dykes DD, Polesky HP. A simple salting out procedure for extracting DNA from human nucleated cells. *Nucleic Acids Res* 1988; 16: 1215.

18. Or R, Kapelushnik J, Naparstek E, *et al.* Second transplantation using allogeneic peripheral blood stem cells in a β-thalassaemia major patient featuring stable mixed chimaerism. *Br J Haematol* 1996; 94: 285–7.

19. Or R, Naparstek E, Cividalli G, Aker M, Engelhard D, Slavin S, Rachmilewitz EA. Bone marrow transplantation in β-thalassemia major: The Israeli experience. *Hemoglobin* 1988; 12: 609–14.

20. Kapelushnik J, Or R, Filon D, Nagler A, Cividalli G, Aker M, Naparstek E, Slavin S, Oppenheim A. Analysis of β-globin mutations shows stable mixed chimerism in patients with thalassemia after bone marrow transplantation. *Blood* 1995; 86: 3241–6.

21. Rund D, Cohen T, Filon D, Dowling CE, Warren TC, Barak I, Rachmilewitz E, Kazazian HH Jr, Oppenheim A. Evolution of a genetic disease in an ethnic isolate: β-thalassemia in the Jews of Kurdistan. *Proc Natl Acad Sci USA* 1991; 88: 310–6.

22. Aker M, Kapelushnik J, Pugatsch T, Naparstek E, Ben-Neria S, Yehuda O, Amar A, Nagler A, Slavin S, Or R. Donor lymphocyte infusions to displace residual host hematopoietic cells after allogeneic bone marrow transplantation for β-thalassemia major. *J Pediat Hematol Oncol* 1998; 20: 1445–8.

23. Pugatsch T, Oppenheim A, Slavin S. Improved single-step PCR assay for sex identification post-allogeneic sex-mismatched BMT. *Bone Marrow Transplant* 1996; 17: 273–5.

24. Slavin S, Nagler A, Naparstek E, Kapelushnik J, Aker M, Cividalli G, Varadi G, Kirschbaum M, Ackerstein A, Samuel S, Amar A, Brautbar C, Ben-Tal O, Eldor A, Or R. Nonmyeloablative stem cell transplantation and cell therapy as an alternative to conventional bone marrow transplantation with lethal cytoreduction for the treatment of malignant and nonmalignant hematologic diseases. *Blood* 1998; 91: 756–63.

25. Grigg A, Bardy P, Byron K, Seymour JH, Szer J. Fludarabine-based non-myeloablative chemotherapy followed by infusion of HLA-identical stem cells for relapsed leukaemia and lymphoma. *Bone Marrow Transplant* 1999; 23: 107–10.

26. Giralt S, Estey E, Albitar M, van Besien K, Rondon G, Anderlini P, O'Brien S, Khouri I, Gajewski J, Mehra R, Claxton D, Andersson B, Beran M, Przepiorka D, Koller C, Kornblau S, Korbling M, Keating M, Kantarjian H, Champlin R. Engraftment of allogeneic hematopoietic progenitor cells with purine analog-containing chemotherapy harnessing graft-versus-leukemia without myeloablative therapy. *Blood* 1997; 89: 4531–6.

27. Nagler A. Ackerstein A, Kapelushnik J, Or R, Naparstek E, Slavin S. Donor lymphocyte infusion post-non-myeloablative allogeneic peripheral blood stem cell transplantation for chronic granulomatous disease. *Bone Marrow Transplant* 1999; 24: 339–42.

28. Akioka S, Itoh H, Ueda I, Matsumoto Y, Iwami H, Tsunamoto K, Hibi S, Todo S, Sawada T, Imashuku S. Donor lymphocyte infusion at unstable mixed chimerism in an allogeneic BMT recipient for chronic granulomatous disease. *Bone Marrow Transplant* 1998; 22: 609–11.

29. Khouri IF, Keating M, Korbling M, Przepiorka D, Anderlini P, O'Brien S, Giralt S, Ippoliti C, von Wolff B, Gajewski J, Donato M, Claxton D, Ueno N, Andersson B, Gee A, Champlin R. Transplant lite: induction of graft-versus malignancy using fludarabine-based nonablative chemotherapy and allogeneic blood progenitor-cell transplantation as treatment for lymphoid malignancies. *J Clin Oncol* 1998; 16: 2817–24.

30. Champlin R, Khouri I, Giralt S. Use of nonmyeloablative preparative regimens for allogeneic blood stem cell transplantation: induction of graft-vs-malignancy as treatment for malignant diseases. *J Clin Apheresis* 1999; 14: 45–9.

31. Kapelushnik J, Or R, Slavin S, Nagler A. Case report. A fludarabine-based protocol for bone marrow transplantation in Fanconi's anemia. *Bone Marrow Transplant* 1997; 20: 1109–10.

32. Slavin S. Treatment of life threatening autoimmune diseases with myeloablative doses of immunosuppressive agents and autologous bone marrow transplantation – rationale and experimental background. *Bone Marrow Transplant* 1993; 12: 85–8.

33. Slavin S. Successful treatment of autoimmune disease in (NZB/NZW)F1 female mice by using fractionated total lymphoid irradiation. *Proc Natl Acad Sci USA* 1979; 76: 5274–6.

Complications of non-myeloablative stem cell transplantation

S Giralt

Introduction

Although the use of non-myeloablative stem cell transplantation (NST) is increasing in frequency[1] NST should still be considered an investigational procedure. The use of NST should be limited to carefully prepared protocols carried out at transplant centers with extensive allografting experience. Current experience continues to be relatively limited and the potential for serious complications exist. In this chapter the spectrum of complications associated with NST is reviewed based on the experience from the first generation trials carried out at the University of Texas M. D. Anderson Cancer Center (MDACC). The types of complications associated with NST include those resulting from the transplant procedure itself, those related to the non-myeloablative conditioning regimen, and those that depend on the recipient (see Table 1).

Toxicity

Although the regimens used for NST are less intensive and less toxic than those used in conventional allogeneic transplantation they are still associated with toxicities inherent to each agent used. Thus for most 'non-myeloablative'

Table 1. Potential complications of NST

Complications due to transplant procedure	Drug toxicity
	Infection
	Graft rejection
	GVHD
	Immunodeficiency
	Recurrence
	Secondary malignancies
Complications particular to non-ablative regimens	Early or late autologous reconstitution
	GVHD after DLI or immunosuppression withdrawal
	Mixed chimerism
Complications from co-morbidities	More frequent infections
	More intercurrent medical events
	Higher risk of drug toxicities

Table 2. Toxicities of commonly used chemotherapy agents in NST

Drug	Doses used in NST	Toxicities
Fludarabine	20–30 mg/m^2 x 4–6 days	Neurotoxicity
Cladribine	4–12 mg/m^2 x 4–5 days	Neurotoxicity
Idarubicin	12 mg/m^2 x 3 days	Mucositis
		Cardiotoxicity
Cytarabine	1–2 g/m^2 x 4–5 days	Mucositis
		Neurotoxicity
Cyclophosphamide	300–1000 mg/m^2 x 3–5 days	Cystitis
Busulfan	8 mg/kg	Veno-occlusive disease
		Pneumonitis
Melphalan	100–180 mg/m^2	Mucositis
		Diarrhea
Tacrolimus	Adjusted to keep levels between 5–10 ng/dl	Nephrotoxicity
		Neurotoxicity
Cyclosporine	Adjusted to keep levels between 100–300 ng/dl	Nephrotoxicity
		Neurotoxicity
Steroids	Various	Myopathy
		Diabetes
		Cataracts
Antithymocyte globulin (ATG)	10–40 mg/kg	Hypersensitivity
		Serum sickness

regimens some degree of myelosuppression is seen and, depending on the combination of drugs, other toxicities can also be observed (Table 2).[2]

The non-myeloablative regimens of particular interest include
- fludarabine/cyclophosphamide (FC) pioneered at MDACC[3] and National Institute of Health[4]
- regimens using low-dose total body irradiation (TBI) as pioneered by the Seattle group or
- regimens using thymic irradiation as used in Boston.[5,6]

These regimens have little acute toxicity and are associated with minimal myelosuppression; patients rarely require transfusion support. The Seattle regimen has been administered almost completely in the outpatient setting.[5] Longer follow up will be required to assess the possible long-term complications of NST such as secondary malignancies, thyroid dysfunction, cataracts, and other effects associated with higher doses of radiation.[7]

Careful assessment of all new regimens is warranted. The combination of cladribine and melphalan was studied at MDACC following successful use of the combination of cladribine and cytarabine in the NST setting.[8–11] A dose below the maximum tolerated dose for each drug was chosen, however, the combination resulted in an unacceptably high incidence of renal failure in 3 of 4 patients in untreated first relapse of acute myelogenous leukemia, prompting the closure of this study arm.[12] The reason for this increased toxicity is un-known but could be due to synergistic damage on the kidney from both melphalan and cladribine in the presence of tacrolimus which is a known nephrotoxin.[13]

Patients receiving NST are typically older and more debilitated than patients receiving conventional allogeneic transplants and thus are more likely to de-velop complications even with standard doses of chemotherapy. These complications will tend to be more severe, and associated with more morbid-ity, than in younger patients.[14] Although non-ablative regimens are devised to take these factors into account, even the best tolerated chemotherapy agents can be associated with fatal toxicities in the elderly patient.

Notwithstanding the above, the truly non-ablative regimens reported to date have been associated with minimal toxicity as can be seen in Table 3. With reduced intensity conditioning regimens, toxicity has been acceptable in older patients with good performance status and no active infections.

Graft-versus-host disease (GVHD)

Once donor cells engraft, the development of GVHD is a possibility. Clinical experience and animal models all demonstrate the importance of tissue dam-age and cytokines as a triggering event for GVHD.[15–17] Life-threatening GVHD can still occur without any chemotherapy (as happens after donor lymphocyte infusion [DLI] or transfusion associated GVHD).[18,19] Likewise, even low lev-els of donor cell chimerism can cause GVHD.[20]

Experience from our center and others seems to suggest that the incidence and severity of GVHD may be less after truly non-ablative preparative regimens. Whereas, reduced-intensity conditioning regimens seem to be associated with the same incidence of GVHD as myeloablative regimens (Table 4). However,

Table 3. Incidence of Grade III or IV Bearman toxicities after non-ablative or reduced-intensity preparative regimens

Preparative regimen	Grade III–IV Bearman toxicity (organ site involved)
Fludarabine/idarubicin/cytarabine	3–5% heart, lung, liver, myelosuppression
FC	< 5% heart, lung, liver, myelosuppression
200 cGy TBI	Minimal myelosuppression
Fludarabine/cyclophosphamide/thymic XRT	Myelosuppression, mucositis
Fludarabine/busulfan/ATG	5% liver
Fludarabine/melphalan	5–10% liver, lung, kidney, heart
Cladribine/melphalan	50% kidney, liver, lung

Table 4. Incidence of acute GVHD according to regimen intensity and donor disparity

	% Grade II–IV	% Grade III–IV	GVHD deaths
FLAG-ida (6/6 related)			
$n = 29$	17	10	1
FLAG-ida (5/6 related)			
$n = 9$	44	11	1
Fludarabine/melphalan (6/6 related)			
$n = 38$	29	13	5
Fludarabine/melphalan (matched unrelated donor)			
$n = 39$	51	26	12

it is possible that for patients who would normally be eligible for a conventional transplant, the risk and severity of GVHD may be lower following NST or reduced-intensity conditioning. This issue can only be addressed within the confines of carefully designed prospective trials comparing conventional myeloablative conditioning with reduced-intensity and non-myeloablative conditioning regimens.

Responses to first-line NST occur in about 50% of patients, with another 25% of patients responding to second line therapy (Table 5). As with conventional myeloablative therapies the incidence and severity of acute GVHD increases with donor–recipient disparity.

Chronic GVHD represents an important cause of morbidity and mortality after conventional myeloablative conditioning. NST may reduce the incidence of chronic GVHD by reducing the incidence of acute GVHD, however, this remains to be proven. Our experience to date suggests that the manifestation of chronic GVHD after NST and reduced-conditioning regimens parallels that seen after conventional myeloablative therapies, with a similar level of response to immunosuppressive therapy also observed (Table 6). Factors that are known to affect the occurrence of chronic GVHD such as donor compatibility, donor sex, use of peripheral blood stem cells, and methods of GVHD prophylaxis will probably play a role in the occurrence of chronic GVHD after NST. These factors will need to be carefully studied to devise the optimal NST strategy for each particular patient and disease.[21–23]

Table 5. Chronic GVHD after non-ablative and reduced-intensity conditioning

	FLAG-ida	Fludarabine/melphalan
% with chronic GVHD	26	53
% with chronic GVHD of limited stage	25	30
% with chronic GVHD of extensive stage	75	70
Tissue involvement	Skin/liver/mucosa 5/6	Skin/liver/mucosa 7/24
	Lung 1/6	Lung 2/24
		Multiorgan 8/24
% Response to first line therapy	57	62
Chronic GVHD deaths	0	3

Table 6. Acute GVHD after non-ablative and reduced-intensity conditioning – response to steroid therapy

	Truly non-ablative therapy	Reduced-intensity conditioning
	FLAG-ida	Fludarabine/melphalan
n	31	66
Number with Grade II–IV GVHD	9	30
% Response to first-line therapy	55	53
Number receiving second-line therapy	4	12
% Response to second-line therapy	25	25
GVHD deaths	3	15

Graft rejection

Graft rejection is a relatively rare occurrence after conventional myeloablative therapy and allogeneic transplantation using unmanipulated bone marrow or stem cells from an HLA identical sibling donor.[24] HLA disparity and T-cell depletion increase the risk of graft rejection to 10–20%. Increasing the intensity of the preparative regimen, or adding more immunosuppressive therapy (such as ATG) has overcome this increased risk of rejection in many studies.[25–28] Therefore the use of less intensive conditioning could be associated with a higher risk of graft rejection.

Graft rejection rates in NST studies so far have ranged from < 5% for some reduced-intensity conditioning regimens to 20% in patients receiving truly non-ablative regimens such as FC or low dose TBI.[1] The risk of graft rejection after non-ablative or reduced-intensity conditioning will probably depend on the degree of donor–recipient compatibility, the underlying disease, and the immune competence of the patient prior to transplant as determined by the disease and the degree of prior therapy. Thus, the intensity of the preparative regimen used should be adjusted to account for the disease being treated, its sensitivity to immune manipulation, and the degree of donor–recipient disparity (Figure 1). T cell chimerism during the first month of transplant and a history of a prior autologous transplant have been reported to predict a higher likelihood of > 50% donor T-cells by day 28 which in turn translates into a higher risk of GVHD and a lower risk of rejection.[29]

Autologous reconstitution generally occurs in patients who reject their graft. However, autologous reconstitution relies on the existence of a functional pool of recipient stem cells that have not been damaged by the disease, prior therapy, or graft versus hematopoietic tissue that could have resulted from transient donor cell engraftment. Of note, all patients with chronic myeloid leukemia (CML) that we and others have treated with NST recovered autologous

143

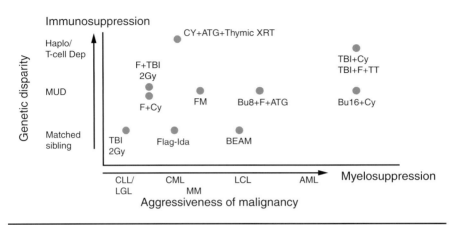

Figure 1. A continuum of non-myeloablative and reduced intensity conditioning regimens

hematopoiesis after graft rejection. In contrast, one patient with refractory acute myeloid leukemia (AML) who rejected their graft had profound cytopenia lasting more than 30 days and failed to respond to a second non-ablative regimen followed by a second infusion of donor stem cells. This suggests that in patients with a poor autologous reserve (as would be expected in a patient with refractory leukemia, or a heavily pretreated patient) autologous reconstitution may not be possible, and subsequent infusions of more donor cells may be unsuccessful because of sensitization.

The issue of sensitization will require careful study but, based on the information obtained from the first generation trials, patients failing NST may have a higher risk of graft failure during a subsequent myeloablative transplant if the original donor is used. In our initial studies, patients who relapsed after receiving FLAG-ida or cladribine/ara-C as conditioning underwent a second transplant using the original donor. For the second transplant patients were conditioned with either high-dose melphalan or busulfan/cyclophosphamide. Two of the 8 patients who underwent this procedure failed to engraft. Likewise, using the same donor for a conventional transplant and NST when applied as salvage therapy for patients not responding to the first transplant may result in an increased risk of graft rejection. This is particularly relevant in the non HLA-identical situation. Two of 5 patients who received either a truly non-ablative regimen or reduced-intensity conditioning for relapse after a myeloablative regimen failed to engraft and had autologous reconstitution (only after infusion of previously stored autologous stem cells in one patient). Therefore, use of an alternative donor may be warranted if a non-ablative regimen is contemplated in a patient who has been sensitized to a previous donor.

Infection

Truly non-ablative regimens should result in limited myelosuppression, and thus should be associated with a lower risk of infectious complications. It has also been postulated that since non-ablative regimens are associated with persistent autologous immune cells, the immune deficiency that typically characterizes the early and mid post-transplant period will be less severe, and thus the risk of viral and fungal infection may be lower. This has not been shown to be the case to date. This lack of effect on incidence of infection may be partly related to the type of patients who have so far undergone NST, and partly to the fact that these patients remain profoundly immunodeficient because of immunosuppressive therapy given to prevent GVHD, or to the presence of GVHD itself. Our experience using truly non-ablative regimens and reduced-intensity conditioning regimens in myeloid leukemias suggests that the spectrum of infectious complications seen following NST is similar to that seen after conventional myeloablative regimens (Table 7). A formal analysis comparing the incidence of various infectious complications post non-ablative, reduced-intensity and myeloablative conditioning is planned.

Recurrence

Dose intensity of TBI has been shown to be important in reducing the risk of relapse after allogeneic transplantation.[30,31] Therefore, relapse rates after reduced-intensity or non-ablative conditioning will be increased because of the induced dose intensity of TBI. However, as long as the increase in relapse rate can be managed successfully (using immunosuppression withdrawal or DLI), it need not negatively impact on survival.

Thirty-one of 45 patients with AML/myelodysplastic syndrome failed to respond to or relapsed after NST. All patients failed to respond to immunosuppression withdrawal, and no patient responded to DLI with or without chemotherapy. Only 2 of 6 patients undergoing a second stem cell transplant with reduced-intensity conditioning obtained long term disease control. Of 4

Table 7. Infectious complication after NST

	FLAG-ida	Fludarabine/melphalan
n	26/45	37/83
Bacteria	21	36
Viral	11	22
Fungus	5	5

patients with CML who were transplanted during their chronic phase and who achieved donor cell engraftment, 2 have relapsed; 1 responded to immunosuppression withdrawal and DLI, the other failed to respond to DLI.

Co-morbid conditions

Older patients have a higher frequency of co-morbidities and these may contribute to complications post-transplant. Although to date our experience is relatively limited we have seen 3 patients with viscus perforation (2 diverticuli, 1 peptic ulcer); 3 with hypertensive central nervous system bleeds and 1 who developed angina. These complications were all secondary to pre-existing medical conditions. Other common complications seen in older patients include steroid myopathy, steroid-induced diabetes mellitus, and drug-induced renal dysfunction.

In summary

NST should not be viewed as an 'easy' form of allografting. This procedure, although well-tolerated in patients who are poor candidates for conventional myeloablative therapies, is still associated with complications that can be severe and life-threatening. Immune-manipulation to prevent relapse or enhance donor cell engraftment can result in serious life-threatening GVHD, infectious complications and serious morbidity and mortality. Therefore, although NST is a new approach that could potentially increase the number of indications and therefore the number of patients that could be successfully treated with an allogeneic transplant, it should still be considered an investigational technique and its use limited to protocol studies.

References

1. Giralt S. Non-myeloablative stem cell transplantation: lessons from the first generation trials. *Leuk Lymphoma Updates* 1999; 2: 4–7.

2. Chabner B, Myers C. Clinical pharmacology of cancer chemotherapy. In *Cancer Principles and Practice of Oncology*. 3rd Edition. DeVita V, Hellman S, Rosenberg S (eds). J B Lipincott, Philadelphia, 1989.

3. Khouri I, Keating M, Korbling M, Przepiorka D, Anderlini P, O'Brien S, Giralt S, Ippoliti C, von Wolff B, Gajewski J, Donato M, Claxton D, Ueno N, Andersson B, Gee A, Champlin R. Transplant lite: induction of graft-versus-malignancy using fludarabine-based nonablative chemotherapy and allogeneic blood progenitor-cell transplantation as treatment for lymphoid malignancies. *J Clin Oncol* 1998; 16: 2817–24.

4. Childs R, Contentin N, Cleve E, Contentin N, Clave E, Bahceci E, Hensel N, Boland C, Pomper G, Read EJ, Leitman S, Dunbar C, Young NS, Barrett AJ. Reduced toxicity and transplant related mortality (TRM) following non-myeloablative allogeneic peripheral blood stem cell transplantation for malignant disease. *Blood* 1999; 94(Suppl. 1): 393.

5. McSweeney P, Niederwieser D, Shizuru J, Molina A, Wagner J, Minor S, Radich J, Chauncey T, Hegenbart U, Maloney D, Nash R, Sandmaier B, Blume K, Storb R. Outpatient allografting with minimally myelosuppressive immunosuppressive conditioning of low dose TBI and postgrafting cyclosporine (CSP) and mycophenolate mofetil (MMF). *Blood* 1999; 94(Suppl. 1): 393.

6. Spitzer T, McAfee S, Sackstein R, *et al*. Induction of mixed chimerism and potent anti-tumor responses following non-myeloablative conditioning therapy and HLA-matched and mismatched donor bone marrow transplantation (BMT) for refractory hematologic malignancies. *Blood* 1998; 92(Suppl. 1): 519.

7. Deeg H. Delayed complications and long term effects after bone marrow transplantation. *Bone Marrow Transplant* 1990; 4: 641–57.

8. Giralt S, Estey E, Albitar M, van Besien K, Rondon G, Anderlini P, O'Brien S, Khouri I, Gajewski J, Mehra R, Claxton D, Andersson B, Beran M, Przepiorka D, Koller C, Kornblau S, Korbling M, Keating M, Kantarjian H, Champlin R. Engraftment of allogeneic hematopoieetic progenitor cells with purine analog-containing chemotherapy: Harnessing graft-versus-leukemia without myeloablative therapy. *Blood* 1997; 89: 4531–6.

9. Sarosy G, Leyland-Jones B, Soochan P, Cheson B. The systemic administration of intravenous melphalan. *J Clin Oncol* 1988; 6: 1768–82.

10. Vahdat L, Wong E, Wile M, Rosenblum M, Foley KM, Warrell RP Jr. Therapeutic and neurotoxic effects of 2-chlorodeoxyadenosine in adults with acute myeloid leukemia. *Blood* 1994; 84: 3429–34.

11. Kornblau S, Gandhi V, Andreeff M, Beran M, Kantarjian HM, Koller CA, O'Brien S, Plunkett W, Estey E. Clinical and laboratory studies of 2-chlorodeoxyadenosine + cytosine arabinoside for relapsed or refractory acute myelogenous leukemia in adults. *Leukemia* 1996; 10: 1563–9.

12. Giralt S, Khouri I, Braunschweig I, Ippolitti C, Claxton D, Donato M, Cohen A, Davis M, Andersson B, Anderlini P, Gajewski J, Kornblau S, Andreeff M, Przepiorka D, Ueno N, Molldrem J, Champlin R. Melphalan and purine analog containing preparative regimens: less intensive conditioning for patients with hematologoic malignancies undergoing allogeneic progenitor cell transplantation. *Blood* 1999; 94 (Suppl. 1): 564.

13. Hooks M. Tacrolimus, a new immunosuppressant – review of the literature. *Ann Pharmacol* 1994; 28: 501–11.

14. Baducci L, Corcoran M. Antineoplastic chemotherapy of the older cancer patient. *Hematol Oncol Clin N America* 2000; 14: 193–212.

15. Ferrara J, Deeg H. Mechanisms of disease: graft versus host disease. *N Engl J Med* 1991; 324: 667–74.

16. Holler E, Kolb H, Eissner G, *et al.* Cytokines in GvH and GvL. *Bone Marrow Transplant* 1998; 22 (Suppl. 4): S3–S6.

17. Holler E, Ertl B, Hintermeier-Knabe R, Roncarolo MG, Eissner G, Mayer F, Fraunberger P, Behrends U, Pfannes W, Kolb HJ, Wilmanns W. Inflammatory reactions induced by pre-transplant conditioning - an alternative target for modulation of acute GvHD and complications following allogeneic bone marrow transplantation? *Leuk Lymphoma* 1997; 25: 217–24.

18. Kolb H, Schattenberg A, Goldman J, Hertenstein B, Jacobsen N, Arcese W, Ljungman P, Ferrant A, Verdonck L, Niederwieser D. Graft-vs-leukemia effect of donor lymphocyte transfusions in marrow grafted patients. *Blood* 1995; 86: 2041–50.

19. Orlin J, Ellis M. Transfusion associated graft versus host disease. *Curr Opin Hematol* 1997; 4: 442–8.

20. Porter D, Connors JM, Van Deerlin VM, Duffy KM, McGarigle C, Saidman SL, Leonard DG, Antin JH. Graft-versus-tumor induction with donor leukocyte infusions as primary therapy for patients with malignancies. *J Clin Oncol* 1999; 17: 1234–43.

21. Parkman R. Chronic graft-versus-host-disease. *Curr Opin Hematol* 1998; 5: 22–5.

22. Sullivan K, Shulman H, Storb R, Weiden PL, Witherspoon RP, McDonald GB, Schubert MM, Atkinson K, Thomas ED. Chronic graft-versus-host disease in 52 patients; adverse natural course and successful treatment with combination immunosuppression. *Blood* 1981; 2: 267–76.

23. Urbano-izpizua A, Garcia-Conde J, Brunet S, Hernandez F, Sanz G, Petit J, Bargay J, Figuera A, Rovira M, Solano C, Ojeda E, de la Rubia J, Rozman C. High incidence of chronic graft-versus-host-disease after allogeneic peripheral blood progenitor cell transplantation. *Haematologica* 1997; 82: 683–9.

24. Storb R, Prentice R, Thomas E, Appelbaum FR, Deeg HJ, Doney K, Fefer A, Goodell BW, Mickelson E, Stewart P. Factors associated with graft rejection after HLA-identical marrow transplantation for aplastic anemia. *Br J Haematol* 1983; 55: 573–5.

25. Hale G, Zhang M, Bunjes D, Prentice HG, Spence D, Horowitz MM, Barrett AJ, Waldmann H. Improving the outcome of bone marrow transplantation by using CD52 monoclonal antibodies to prevent graft-versus-host disease and graft rejection. *Blood* 1998; 92: 4581–9.

26. Rufer N, Starobinski M, Chapuis B, Gratwohl A, Jeannet M, Helg C, Roosnek E. Clinical consequences of sensitisation to minor histocompatibility antigens before allogeneic bone marrow transplantation. *Bone Marrow Transplant* 1998; 22: 895–8.

27. Molina A, McSweeney P, Maloney D, Sandmaier B, Wagner JL, Nash R, Chauncey T, Bryant E, Storb R. Degree of early donor T-cell chimerism predicts GVHD and graft rejection in patients with nonmyeloablative hematopoietic stem cell allografts. *Blood* 1999; 94: 394a.

Current and future approaches of hematopoietic tumor specific cellular therapy

E Goulmy

Minor histocompatibility antigens (mHags) are peptides from low poly-morphic intracellular proteins.[1] These proteins are digested within the cytosol and peptides from them can bind to major histocompatability complex (MHC) class I molecules and be presented at the cell surface. Intracellular proteins that differ in their amino acid sequence result in different fragments that may lead to MHC restricted T cell activation.

The classical definition of mHags originates from the observations of cellular alloimmune responses in recipients of MHC identical transplants.[2] mHag specific T cells isolated from patients primed *in vivo* by HLA identical stem cell transplantation (SCT) were used to study the various immunobiological characteristics of human mHags (Table 1).

The mHag specific T cell clones have also been used for the identification of the chemical nature of the mHags. Since mHags are recognized by T cells in association with MHC molecules, one approach is to isolate these antigen from their respective MHC molecules. The application of microcapillary high-performance liquid chromatography (HPLC) electrospray ionization tandem mass spectrometry was applied for the detection of these minor H antigen (mH) non-abundant peptides among a pool of MHC-bound peptides.[3] Using the latter methodology, we have chemically identified the mH peptide ligands of some of our local T cell clones[4–8] (Table 2). As illustrated in Table 2, the Y chromosome and autosomal genes encode mHags.

mHag disparities between HLA matched stem cell donors and recipients may induce post-SCT alloresponses participating in both graft-versus-host disease (GVHD) and graft-versus-leukemia (GVL) reactions. With regard to the postulated mHag T cell reactivities involved in the GVL effect, investigation of

Table 1. Some characteristics of human mHags

- Non-MHC encoded transplantation antigens
- Recognition by MHC restricted T cells
- Variable phenotype frequencies
- Mendelian segregation
- Restricted or broad tissue distribution

Table 2. Human mHags

mHags	Genes	Chromosomes	AA sequences	Restriction molecules	Tissue distribution
H-Y	SMCY	Y	FIDSYICQV	HLA-A2	broad
H-Y	SMCY	Y	SPSVDKARAEL	HLA-B7	broad
H-Y	DFFRY	Y	IVDCLTEMY	HLA-A1	broad
HA-1	?	19	VLHDDLLEA	HLA-A2	restricted
HA-2	myosin	?	VIGEVSVSV	HLA-A2	restricted

functional HLA–mHag peptide ligand membrane expression is crucial. Our analyses of the membrane expression of a limited number of mHags using our mHag specific cytotoxic T cell clones revealed that all mHags investigated (i.e. H-Y and HA-1 to HA-5) are expressed on hematopoietic progenitor cells,[9] on clonogenic leukemic precursor cells[10] and on circulating leukemic cells of lymphocytic and myeloid origin.[11] However, the tissue expression of some mHags (i.e. HA-1 and HA-2) is limited to the hematopoietic system only, whereas other mHags (i.e. H-Y and HA-3) are ubiquitously expressed.[12]

Absence of both mHag cytotoxic and helper T cell alloreactivities post-HLA-matched SCT may result in relapse of leukemia (Table 3). We therefore propose using adoptive immunotherapy with cytotoxic T cells (CTLs) specific for hematopoietic, system specific mHags. This is, in principle, similar to immunotherapy with donor buffycoat cells. Yet, adoptive immunotherapy with CTLs specific for hematopoietic-system-restricted mHags is patient- and hematopoietic-system specific. The use of mHag specific CTLs as adoptive immunotherapy of leukemia is based on three of the known characteristics of human mHag, i.e.
- MHC restricted recognition by T cells
- immunogenic polymorphism beyond HLA
- restricted tissue distribution i.e. expression only on hematopoietic cells including leukemic cells and their progenitors.

Evidently, the mHags with restricted tissue distribution are candidates for adoptive immunotherapy of leukemia. Our candidates to date are mHag HA-1 and

Table 3. Synergistic effects of mHag specific CTL/Th cells on GVHD and GVL in HLA matched SCT

Anti-host T cell activities	Status GVHD/relapse	
	no / relapse	acute grade II or more
CTL and Th	2	10
CTL alone	2	2
Th alone	0	1
no CTL, no Th	3/3	0

HA-2, of which their hematopoietic system restricted expression has been clearly demonstrated earlier.[10]

We developed in *vitro* Good Manufacturing Practice (GMP) graded protocols of HA-1 and HA-2 specific CTLs for adoptive immunotherapy of relapsed leukemia after HLA matched, HA-1 and/or HA-2 mismatched SCT.[13] A phase I/II study has been initiated at our academic center. Before SCT, we type all HLA-A2 positive SCT patients and their potential HLA matched SCT donors-for the mHags HA-1 and HA-2. Typing for HA-1 can be carried out on DNA samples. The genomic identification of the mHag HA-1 locus is done by allele specific PCR.[14] The HA-1 locus has two alleles – the HA-1^H and the HA-1^R alleles. These alleles differ by two nucleotides which results in a single amino acid substitution.[7] Typing for mHag HA-2 is to date still carried out using cell mediated lympholysis with mHag HA-2 specific CTLs. Although we have identified the HA-2 peptide sequence,[2] we have not yet characterized the HA-2 coding region. Thus, for our clinical trial, for example in case we identified an HA-1 allelic difference between an HLA-A2 matched patient and donor (i.e. donor HA-1$^{R/R}$, patient HA-1$^{H/R}$ or HA-1$^{H/H}$), we generate mHag HA-1^H peptide specific CTLs *ex vivo* from the mHag HA-1$^{R/R}$ SCT donor. The generation of these *ex vivo* mHag specific CTLs, their expansion kinetics and specificity testing are described in detail elsewhere.[11] Upon transfusion, the mHag HA-1^H specific CTL will eliminate the HA-1^H patient's hematopoietic cells including the patient's leukemic cells. Based on the use of mHag with restricted expression to the hematopoietic cell-lineage, the patient's non-hematopoietic cells and tissues as well as the mHag HA-1$^{R/R}$ marrow of the original stem cell donor, will be spared.

Leukemia patients with advanced relapsed disease who are resistant to treatment with donor buffy coat cells, are eligible for our phase I/II trial. In case of relapse, the SCT donor derived mHag specific CTLs will be infused when donor engraftment has reached $\geq 50\%$. The studies will optionally use transduction of CTLs with suicide genes. As mentioned earlier, we established the *in vitro* generation of HLA-A2 HA-1 and HA-2 specific CTLs. To broaden the number of relapsed patients eligible for mHag specific CTL adoptive therapy, we are currently investigating whether other (i.e. not HLA-A2) HLA alleles also bind the HA-1 and/or HA-2 peptides. Moreover, the HA-1 and HA-2 genes will be sequenced enabling the search for additional polymorphism(s) in the population.

As the number of HLA mismatched SCTs increases, our future focus will be the use of hematopoietic system specific mHags in the context of HLA partially mismatched SCT for the treatment of leukemia relapse. Here, the patient's mismatched HLA molecules, which are absent in the SCT donor, will be used as the target and the antigen-presenting molecule for hematopoietic system specific mHags. Immunotherapy with CTLs directed at a patient's allo-HLA hematopoietic specific mHags should produce *in vivo* results identical to those described above for the HLA matched mHag mismatched protocol.

In summary

Hematopoietic system specific mHags can serve as ingredients for adoptive immunotherapy of relapsed hematologic malignancies in both HLA matched and HLA mismatched SCT. In the former setting, the mHags mismatch is used as a target molecule; in the latter setting the HLA mismatch combined with hematopoietic mHags is used as a target molecule for hematopoietic tumor specific cellular immunotherapy.

References

1. Rötzschke O, Falk K, Wallny HJ, Faath S, Rammensee HG. Characterization of naturally occurring minor histocompatibility peptides including H-4 and H-Y. *Science* 1989; 249: 283–7.

2. Goulmy E. Human minor histocompatibility antigens. *Curr Opin Immunol* 1996; 8: 75–81.

3. Hunt DF, Henderson RA, Shabanowicz J, Sakaguchi K, Michel H, Sevilir N, Cox A, Appella E, Engelhard VH. Characterization of peptides bound to class I MHC molecule HLA-A2.1 by mass spectrometry. *Science* 1992; 255: 1261–3.

4. den Haan JM, Sherman NE, Blokland E, Huczko E, Koning F, Drijfhout JW, Skipper J, Shabanowitz J, Hunt DF, Engeldhard VH, Goulmy E. Identification of a graft versus host disease-associated human minor histocompatibility antigen. *Science* 1995; 268: 1467–80.

5. Wang W, Meadows LR, den Haan JM, Sherman NE, Chen Y, Blokland E, Shabanowitz J, Agulnik AI, Hendrickson RC, Bishop C, Hunt DF, Goulmy E, Engelhard VH. Human H-Y: a male-specific histocompatibility antigen derived from the SMCY protein. *Science* 1995; 269:1588–90.

6. Meadows L, Wang W, den Haan JM, Blokland E, Reinhardus C, Drijfhout JW, Shabanowitz J, Pierce R, Agulnik AI, Bishop CE, Hunt DF, Goulmy E, Engelhard VH. The HLA-A*0201-restricted H-Y antigen contains a post-translationally modified cysteine that significantly affects T cell recognition. *Immunity* 1997; 6: 273–81.

7. den Haan JM, Meadows LM, Wang W, Pool J, Blokland E, Bischop TL, Reinhardus C, Shabanowitz J, Offringa R, Hunt DF, Engelhard VH, Goulmy E. The minor histocompatibility antigen HA-1: a diallelic gene with a single amino acid polymorphism. *Science* 1998; 279: 1054–7.

8. Pierce RA, Field ED, den Haan JMM, Marto JA, Wang W, Frost LM, Blokland E, Reinhardus C, Shabanowitz J, Hunt DF, Goulmy E, Engelhard VH. The HLA-A*0101-restricted HY minor Histocompatibility antigen originates from DFFRY and contains a cysteinylated cysteine residue as identified by a novel mass spectrometric technique. *J Immunol* 1999; 163: 6360–4.

9. Marijt WAF, Veenhof WFJ, Goulmy E, Willemze R, van Rood JJ, Falkenburg JHF. Minor histocompatibility antigen HA-1, -2, -4 and HY specific cytotoxic T cell clones inhibit human hematopoietic progenitor cell growth by a mechanism that is dependent on direct cell–cell contact. *Blood* 1993; 82: 3778–85.

10. Falkenburg F, Goselink H, van der Harst D, van Luxemburg-Heijst S, Kooy-Winkelaar Y, Faber L, de Kroon J, Brand A, Fibbe W, Willemze R, Goulmy E. Growth inhibition of clonogenic leukemic precursor cells by minor histocompatibility antigen specific cytotoxic T lymphocytes. *J Exp Med* 1991; 174: 27–33.

11. van der Harst D, Goulmy E, Falkenburg JHF, Kooij-Winkelaar Y, van Luxemburg-Heijs SAP, Goselink HM, Brand A. Recognition of minor histocompatibility antigens on lymphocytic and myeloid leukemic cells by cytotoxic T cell clones. *Blood* 1994; 83: 1060–6.

12. de Bueger M, Bakker A, van Rood JJ, van der Woude F, Goulmy E. Tissue distribution of human minor Histocompatibility antigen. Ubiquitous versus restricted tissue distribution indicates heterogeneity among human CTLs defined non-MHC antigens. *J Immunol* 1992; 149: 1788–94.

13. Mutis T, Verdijk R, Schrama E, Esendam B, Brand A, Goulmy E. Feasibility of immunotherapy of relapsed leukemia with *ex vivo*-generated cytotoxic T lymphocytes specific for hematopoietic system-restricted minor Histocompatibility antigens. *Blood* 1999; 93; 2336–41.

14. Wilke M, Pool J, den Haan JMM, Goulmy E. Genomic identification of the minor Histocompatibility Antigen HA-1 locus by allele specific PCR. *Tissue Antigens* 1998; 52: 312–7.

Summary and conclusions
S Slavin, S Giralt

Non-myeloablative conditioning is feasible and relatively safe even in heavily treated high-risk patients with a range of indications for stem cell transplantation. Non-myeloablative stem cell transplantation (NST) is associated with minimal procedure-related toxicity and mortality, shorter periods of pancytopenia with minimal or no aplasia and hence reduced consumption of blood products and anti-microbial therapy. NST is therefore well tolerated by patients including those traditionally considered ineligible for allogeneic transplantation because of older age or poor performance status. Stable complete or mixed chimerism can be induced consistently for patients with a matched sibling or matched unrelated donor. Early complete engraftment is observed in most patients but in cases of mixed chimerism, conversion to 100% donor cells can be accomplished by discontinuing cyclosporine (CSA) treatment or by giving an infusion of donor lymphocytes (DLI). The same approach can also be applied to patients whose disease relapses following NST. If rejection of the graft occurs, the patient is likely to have autologous hematopoietic reconstitution. Shorter durations of hospitalization and the possibility of using NST in the outpatient setting may result in improved cost-effectiveness.

Thus, NST may become the procedure of choice for elderly patients in need of bone marrow transplantation. For younger patients, NST may allow effective treatment of patients with a wide range of indications for bone marrow transplantation while reducing the risk of sterility and other late complications including endocrine adenopathies and growth retardation. Once proven to be safe, NST may provide an incentive for clinicians to consider curative rather than palliative treatment at an early stage of disease for both malignant and non-malignant indications.

To further improve the outcome of NST the aims for future studies should be to:
- minimize procedure-related risks by defining the minimum conditioning required for consistent engraftment
- define the optimal conditioning for each disease category for patients with high and low tumor bulks
- focus on improving efficacy and specificity of immunotherapy mediated by donor lymphocytes

- optimize methods for prevention of GVHD in patients with non-malignant diseases
- optimize control of GVHD in patients with malignant disease using minimal post-transplant immunosuppression
- facilitate immunological reconstitution following NST to minimize infectious complications.

We believe that the aforementioned goals can be met by studying innovative ideas in large cooperative groups. Successful phase I and II clinical trials are urgently needed to define optimal NST protocols for each disease category, carried out in transplant centers that will also be committed to carrying out phase III clinical trials comparing NST with conventional myeloablative regimens. NST may the first step in the introduction of smarter anti-cancer modalities that focus on immunotherapy, rather than using more aggressive and hence potentially hazardous chemoradiotherapy. Well-organized prospective multicenter cooperative studies are the only way to develop NST as an optimal therapeutic modality for the treatment of patients in need of bone marrow transplantation.

Index